mind

body

cleanse

mind

body

cleanse

chris james

Vermilion
LONDON

1 3 5 7 9 10 8 6 4 2

Vermilion, an imprint of Ebury Publishing,
20 Vauxhall Bridge Road,
London SW1V 2SA

Vermilion is part of the Penguin Random House group of companies whose
addresses can be found at global.penguinrandomhouse.com

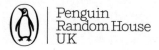

This edition first published in the United Kingdom by Vermilion in 2017

www.penguin.co.uk

A CIP catalogue record for this book is available from the British Library

ISBN 9781785040801

Typeset in India by Integra Software Services Pvt. Ltd, Pondicherry

Printed and bound in Great Britain by Clays Ltd, St Ives PLC

Penguin Random House is committed to a sustainable future for our
business, our readers and our planet. This book is made from
Forest Stewardship Council® certified paper.

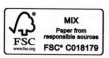

The information in this book has been compiled by way of general guidance
in relation to the specific subjects addressed, but it is not a substitute and not
to be relied on for medical, healthcare, pharmaceutical or other professional
advice on specific circumstances and in specific locations. Please consult
your GP before changing, stopping or starting any medical treatment. So far
as the author is aware the information given is correct and up to date as at
June 2017. Practice, laws and regulations all change, and the reader should
obtain up to date professional advice on any such issue. The author and
the publishers disclaim, as far as the law allows, any liability arising directly
or indirectly from the use, misuse, of the information contained in this book.

I dedicate this book to my late father, Phillip, and my mother, Vivian.

Contents

Before we get started

'For the spiritual warrior
The act of surrender
Consummates a victory
And nothing important is lost'

K. BRADFORD BROWN

The inspiration behind my Mind Body Cleanse journey

I was told not to move. Men encircled me in white coats. I could hear my sister's voice. She was crying beside me. My head had been masking-taped to the hospital bed and I was unable to move my body.

My neck was broken at C2 and C3, dislocated at C3 and C4. One of the men in white coats informed me that if I moved my head and neck I would spend the rest of my life in a wheelchair. My spinal column was resting on an open fracture, the equivalent of a piece of string on a razor blade; one false move and that could have been it. In this moment I came face to face with my own entombment.

Then, in the morphine-induced din, the events of the previous evening began to piece themselves back together. In A&E I was watching myself watch reality. I was back in the grocer's shop, before the first blow had been struck. I was inside the shop, admiring the incredible array of colours from the confectionery counter. A muffled laughter. Then I was walking up to the grocer's shop with my sister, linking arms, busily chatting before it all happened. And then silence. I couldn't see anything for the film of blood that separated me from reality.

I pleaded. I was in a vice-like grip. I was terribly confused. What had I done? Why was this man so furious with me? What had I done to him? Why was he beating me?

'Please no more,' I said.

And then something beautiful happened, unexpectedly. As I started to slip away, everything went quiet.

The beating had come to a premature end. And before that tap on the shoulder, I remember thinking how sorry I felt for my unmoving, juiceless body that I saw lying on the floor from above.

Suddenly, I was able to run out of the shop. I bolted outside into a sea of noise, police sirens and ambulance lights. I held my head above my shoulders in the palms of my hand and ran.

'Can you hear me, Mr James?' somebody asked.

In the years leading up to the assault, I had been living and practising yoga and meditation in India, enjoying a lifestyle that some might think quite unorthodox. I bought antique textiles in Gujarat and Rajasthan and other parts of India. I also designed simple block-print and screen-print sarongs and blankets. In the summer months I sold my wares on the Portobello Road. The stall told a story of adventure and people loved it.

I lived in an old green miner's bus, which I had rescued from an embankment along the Thames in south-west London. I spent the next month making her roadworthy, while my mechanic, Fabrice, taught me how to bypass the fuel line while smoking Gitanes.

The axles were not quite straight so the minibus drove at a slight angle. And from the minibus roof, a chimney protruded out of a wood-burning stove. This was my dream, a real gypsy wagon. I will never forget the look on my father's face when I drove the minibus home. As if all of the thousands of pounds spent on my education had gone up in a cloud of gypsy smoke.

Like this I followed the sun for a few years.

I came into contact with yoga and meditation mainly through curiosity. In India, I was amazed at the enthusiasm with which other Western travellers spoke about yoga. This new world sounded so wonderfully exotic, this was exactly what I was looking for! On a textiles-buying mission in the Himalaya, as I passed through Rishikesh, I went to find a course and a teacher to help guide me.

In the years that followed, I practised yoga and meditation diligently, sometimes for as long as nine hours each day. In retrospect, the time that I spent devoted to the practice of yoga and meditation had been time well spent. The senior orthopedic surgeon later asked me if my spinal column was made of concrete!

In intensive care, I allowed myself to feel my own pain, the full weight of the assault weighing down upon my shoulders; I was powerless, finally. And that's where it happened. I surrendered, but in a way that I had never really surrendered before.

From that day forward I was completely present, in a way that I had never been present in my life before. I felt enriched from my experience.

My neck was rebuilt with bone from my hip, screws and titanium plates. From the moment I was told my prognosis, I knew that I had to win my life back. So, I used all of the breathing, visualisation and meditation techniques that I had learned, and I successfully brought the intelligence back into my body. It was a marathon, of sorts, but when you are determined to win, nothing can stop you.

The medical staff could not believe how quickly I recovered from the assault. And I walked out of the Whittington Hospital in six weeks with a blue-and-white neck-brace collar.

While I cannot be 100 per cent sure whether my recovery can be exclusively attributed the yoga and meditation, I am quite certain that they played a significant part. I was amazed at the power of this humble teaching and I was placed in a unique position to practise it. As I regained movement, I realised that this simple practice worked, so I decided that this is what I wanted to do with my life: to teach yoga and meditation and share this gift with others.

My whole approach to wellness is based on the fundamental aspects of the practice that I discovered in India. I discovered a link between gut health, the practice of cleansing and nutrition, which together with yoga, breathing and meditation created a path for healing and an enlightened approach to being.

All about my Mind Body Cleanse system and my 12-Day Plan

This book explains how the human 'machine' (comprising body, mind and spirit) works in harmony and how you can use my unique detoxifying 12-Day Plan, which forms Part 2 of this book, as a tool to transform your whole self. Working from our knowledge of how the gut operates in the context of the mind, body and spirit combined and how it is the lynchpin for good health, my easy-to-follow, transforming 12-Day Plan includes a challenging, enjoyable and highly rewarding combination of fasting diet, yogic exercise and breathing, meditation and a wealth of healing and health-care tips to do at home. Combined, these will help you to cleanse toxins from your gut, mitigate the effects of stress, become strong, fit and well and heal your Self, creating peak wholeness and happiness, which can have life-long effects.

IF YOU ARE NEW TO YOGA

This book is suitable for everyone, whether you already have knowledge and experience of the issues and yoga techniques or are just starting out. However, if you are a newcomer it is vital to learn the exercises and asanas in a regular (weekly) class under the supervision of an experienced teacher. Then, having learnt the techniques and been taught and coached by a qualified teacher, you can then go on to practise at home on your own – as part of my 12-Day Plan – and avoid unnecessary strain and injury. The style of yoga described in the book is a Hatha and Iyengar mix, which I have adapted for my own clients, and concentrates mainly on inversions, twists and bends, which are the most effective cleansing asanas to use for our purposes.

The yoga sequences set out in this book are not here to substitute weekly yoga classes. But if you are new to yoga, I recommend signing up to an introductory course or booking in some private classes before starting the 12-Day Plan. Home practice can help you to understand your weekly classes at a more profound level, through making practice more regular – even daily – if you possibly can.

'This Cleanse has taught me that my body performs and looks better when I am putting good, healthy foods inside it. All in all it has been a fantastic experience and I've lost a total of 9lbs.'

About this book

If you have picked up this book for the first time, it is likely that you have just taken your first steps towards creating a brand-new you – may I be the first to congratulate you!

I have written this book to guide you and let you know that it really is possible to re-engage with your mind and body in a completely new way.

Planning for the Plan

It's a good idea to read Part I (Mind Body Cleanse: Background) of the book first of all to get an overall understanding of my Mind Body Cleanse ethos and my unique 12-Day Plan, which I want to share with you. Part 1 tells you all the theory you need to know and understand about your own health, including stress, the vital role of your gut in your health, all about the theory behind yoga, meditation, the breath and the preparation you need to do before embarking on the 12-Day Plan. Then you can move on to Part 2 (The 12-Day Plan: Taking Action), reading the overview of the Plan so that you can get a clear idea of what you will be doing on a daily basis and can devise your own approach. For example, you will need to decide on a start date when you can commit to following the Plan as well as possible. Choose 12 days so that the Power Phase (Days 7–9) falls in a period of relative quiet in your schedule – when you haven't got 10 or 15 back-to-back meetings or are doing the Iron Man competition! Part 2 gives you all the practical information you need about how to do the yoga asanas, how to prepare your food and drink every day with some delicious easy recipes and all about the meditations you will be learning. An at-a-glance chart (see page 112) gives you a quick way of checking the order of the exercises in your daily practice.

- Try to be honest and realistic with yourself – to meet your own needs and expectations. That way you will achieve great results.
- Once you decide on your start date, be mindful of the days leading up to it, so that you can prepare yourself mentally. Read through the whole book, so that you can find out what to expect and be prepared for any challenges that may arise.
- It's a good idea to purchase a notebook to take notes as you go along and record your progress. Writing things down will help you lodge everything in your own mind more effectively. At the beginning of

each phase of the 12-Day Plan, write down your goals and make them as specific as possible. This will help them to become real.

■ After the 12 days of the Plan you will feel refreshed, energised and more in control of your life. You will see the physical results of a more toned body, sparkling eyes and glowing skin, and experience the benefits of increased mental clarity and joy.

■ Many people have experienced weight loss by following the 12-Day Plan, but this should not really be your primary motive. The Plan is not just a quick fix that sees you working towards your beach-toned body, only to return to bad habits afterwards. Instead, think of it as being the start of a long-term life plan. To maintain optimum levels of health and vitality I recommend that you carry out the 12-Day Plan every three or four months each year.

'The Cleanse Plan is easy to follow, no excuses for anyone with a busy schedule. You do have time to do this! You won't get bored or hungry. My fridge has never looked so healthy. I am sure my insides reflect this. I would recommend this to anyone.'

As a health professional, I am adamant that everyone should have a healthy body, both inside and out, and it's my intention to get you to think differently about your relationship with food and drink and how you look after yourself on an ongoing basis. You only have one body, so you should treat it with respect and aim to get it into peak condition. Prepare to be amazed by the results of carrying out my 12-Day Plan. But if you have any health concerns, please discuss them with a health practitioner before embarking on the Plan.

PART 1 Mind body cleanse: background

CHAPTER 1

Our health and what affects it

The human health crisis

Human health across the Western world is deteriorating at an alarming rate as can be seen in the increased incidences of cancer, heart disease, liver infection, respiratory ailments and nervous disorders. Even degenerative illnesses that a century ago rarely manifested themselves except in the weak and elderly have now become everyday conditions in the adult population, and sometimes even in the young.

Obesity in the West has increased to epidemic proportions, and some babies are now even being born obese. How has this happened? Is obesity the result of 'poor' genes or is it the result of how genes have expressed themselves through our modern Western lifestyles, through diet, and through our sedentary office-bound lives?

It's a sad state of affairs, but most of our calories are derived from 'food-like' products, processed sugars, white flours, fried ingredients, saturated animal fats, sweet beverages, soda acid bombs, commercial cereals, added sodium, added chemicals – in fact, very little of what goes into our bodies is actually nutritional.

While part of the problem is commercial advertising and the food industry as a whole, the other part of the problem is the continual on-the-go society that we have created for ourselves – we eat mindlessly, without proper thought and consideration – not because we are hungry, as we did in former times, but out of sheer habit and for a whole raft of other reasons. We may eat because we are stressed, we are tired, we are depressed and if we feel lonely – or just because the clock tells us that it's dinnertime. For many of us, sadly, food has actually become a substitute for love.

Moreover, we eat while we are doing other things and this is far from healthy: while watching television, while working at the computer, while talking with others, while driving and on the move. We are not fully conscious of what we are eating and we have lost our connection with our food. We have become mindless eaters.

And yet, the food we eat still becomes a part of us, of who we are. This, in turn, affects our long-term health.

Toxicity: our downfall

The root cause of our human health crisis is a severing of our relationship with the natural order and this has created toxicity in our lives at many different levels. This is driven by our hectic lifestyles, the use of preservatives and additives in food, and also chemically contaminated air and water, damaging electromagnetic fields and the over-use of medical drugs.

Every single person and animal on the planet contains residues of toxic chemicals or metals in their body tissues. It's a fact that 80,000 new chemicals have been introduced since the turn of the twentieth century but most have never been tested for safety or for synergistic actions. The heavy metals that cause the most ill health are lead, mercury, cadmium, arsenic, nickel and aluminium. Chemical toxins include volatile organic compounds (VOCs), solvents (cleaning materials), medications, alcohol, pesticides, herbicides and food additives. Infections and mould toxins (evident in 'sick-building syndrome') are other common sources of toxins.

In the face of our toxic environment in the twenty-first century, and with the reality that all living species contain increasing levels of environmental toxins with widespread biological effects, it is clear that both new research to elucidate the mechanisms by which toxins affect health and novel strategies for systematic seasonal detoxification are needed.

However, the poisoning that stems from environmental pollution and chronic degenerative disease in itself are not given priority in our healthcare system. This is because our current health paradigm evolved from treating acute disease as the main cause of death at the turn of the twentieth century to treating chronic degenerative disease as we enter the twenty-first. Physicians will eventually have to develop the skills necessary to cope with this trend.

So what does all this mean? And what can we do in our daily lives to mitigate the effects of environmental toxins or external toxins and inner toxins created by poor digestion and poorly chosen foods? On top of this you could easily get lost in the vast array of 'detoxification' products in the market place today. It seems that we are being sold a lie.

Toxic exposure

Exposure to toxins comes from two main sources: firstly from our environment (external toxins) and secondly the gut or the breakdown products of our metabolism. Both of these factors can overload our natural detoxification mechanisms.

Symptoms may occur, such as food allergies and sensitivities, PMS, gut problems, skin problems or headaches and if these are left unchecked, more serious conditions can eventually make their presence felt.

Furthermore, when the intestines provide insufficient relief for the metabolism, other organs of elimination must take their place. The kidneys must increasingly eliminate the predominantly acid waste products in the urine; the skin must secrete more waste; and the lungs have to secrete more toxins with the exhaled breath, often assuming an unhealthy, unpleasant odour.

Inner toxicity and our diet

Our inner state of toxicity is further exacerbated by our modern refined diet because it places an extra burden on detoxification systems and our digestive system, through excessive consumption of sugar, high-fructose corn syrup, trans-fatty acids, alcohol, caffeine, aspartame and the various plastics, pathogens, hormones and antibiotics found in our food supply, and excessive quantities of animal protein.

'The only way to
avoid internal and
external toxins might
be to live an ascetic
lifestyle.'

The only way to avoid internal and external toxins might be to live an ascetic lifestyle, eating only wild foods and drinking spring water, complemented by moving our bodies for two or three hours of physical activity daily.

Unfortunately, toxicity cannot be reversed by modern drugs or by Western invasive surgery: the one and only way to counteract self-toxification is by self-detoxification. Fortunately, a systematic cleanse can be done simply, quickly and efficiently using the 12-Day Plan.

YOUR HEALTH IN YOUR HANDS

Many years ago, in my private one-on-one sessions and my yoga classes, I often found myself wishing I had more time to teach all my clients and students what they needed to know to fully embrace optimal health through total body-mind cleansing.

'After the Cleanse
my skin was clearer, I
had lost weight and
encouragingly people
commented on how
well I looked.'

So I first started working with the 12-Day Plan, as it became known, in 2004 with my private clients, who were typically time-poor and stressed, habitually overindulged and under-exercised, often suffering from mental fog and struggling to find a natural solution to achieving optimum levels of health and wellness. This led me to developing a 12-day health system: a combination of cleansing, detoxing food and drink, yoga poses, meditation and breathing that they could do at home in their own time. It started its life in a shoebox with a simple A4 print-out of instructions.

'The 12-Day Plan
was highly effective
and successful and
I soon started to
see my clients lives
transform for the
better.'

The 12-Day Plan was highly effective and successful and I soon started to see my clients lives transform for the better. I saw very unhealthy people become healthy, happy, fulfilled people. My clients told their friends about it and I started to expand the 12-Day Plan into group settings, workshops, master classes and overseas retreats. The feedback was always so positive that I decided to put my discoveries into a book that everybody could use – and what you are reading now is the result.

The 12-Day Plan is appropriate for people who want to enhance their performance in life and in the workplace; or those whose health might need a reset. The objective is for gradual, sustainable change that will endure over time. Once your body is functioning optimally, your system will metabolise more efficiently and you will continue to experience (continued) many positive changes for years to come. My hope is that by following the 12-Day Plan, you are able to bring your body back to its optimal health and greatly increase the quality of your life, both now and in the future.

'Intelligent movement' is a vital component of Mind Body Cleanse using the 12-Day Plan, and is the style that best describes my approach to the activity parts of the Plan (see page 70). In Part 2 you will find a sequence of yoga poses and techniques that will help you to stimulate your metabolism and heal your gut. The many poses, when combined correctly with the breath, can be a great way to reduce stress. Physically, the Mind Body Cleanse sequences promote strength and create flexibility in the soft tissue. Internally, the Mind Body Cleanse sequence stimulates detoxification and metabolism. Mentally, it establishes clarity as well as confidence.

As we progress through the 12 days of the Plan, with every fresh phase I will add in more Mind Body Cleanse poses and techniques to vary your practice and help you progress through the Plan towards a brand-new you! My hope is that, by following the 12-Day Plan, you will bring back your body and mind to its optimum state of health and wellness, which, after all, is your birthright.

'Physically, the Mind Body Cleanse sequences promote strength and create flexibility in the soft tissue. Internally, the Mind Body Cleanse sequence stimulates detoxification and metabolism. Mentally, it establishes clarity as well as confidence.'

The science of wellness

IMPOSSIBLE STANDARDS

We are constantly being bombarded with media images of impossibly perfect standards of beauty and flawless perfection. And even more invasively, in recent times, on our smart phones and electronic devices and via the wellness cult to be seen on Instagram and other social media. This focus on society's perceived beauty causes a preoccupation with the self and an intensely felt need for perfection. However, something sinister lurks beneath the surface – the messages masquerade as wellness, but if you dig a little deeper you will see that they are rotten to their core.

Our culture promotes a standard of beauty that is not only unrealistic, but is potentially harmful, where appearance addiction and damaging body-image issues prevail and become the norm. This message plagues women and, increasingly, men across the globe, especially those in Western cultures. Body-image problems may cause numerous disorders including: depression, eating disorders, self-mutilation, obsessive exercise, anxiety and isolation. It is all totally dehumanising.

We need to redefine what it means to have a healthy relationship with our minds and our bodies.

'The stomach is the centre of life. A hundred diseases are rooted there. Healing always requires the patient's cooperation.'

TRADITIONAL CHINESE MEDICINE

Western medical science is concerned first and foremost with disease, but rarely with health and healthy people. Billions are spent every year on curing the sick, while very little is spent on preventing illness from occurring in the first place. Without diagnostics for good health in place, many danger signs cannot be recognised early on and people cannot protect themselves from illness in time.

'The human body only accepts food that is natural and wholesome.'

In the human body, the large intestine is the organ that has suffered the most abuse from our contemporary lifestyles because it works best only when the other parts of the digestive system are working well and are in balance. Despite human evolution from ape to space traveller, there has been a serious devolution in terms of our diets. The human body only accepts food that is natural and wholesome because the alimentary canal has not adapted and continues to protect itself from this basic dietary fact, meaning that acidosis, hypoxia and inflammation take root. These conditions of imbalance allow germs to breed, tissues to degenerate and other degenerative conditions to develop. And this is what lies at the root of the human health crisis today.

Bringing back alignment

'The body's natural cleansing mechanisms are not designed to deal with the unnatural mess that we have created.'

So how do we bring ourselves back into alignment with our natural state of optimal health and wellbeing? This can only take place by adopting lifestyle changes and, specifically, focusing on the gut, which is the connective stem that links mind and body. However, it is unrealistic to start a new diet and lifestyle before you have got rid of the years of accumulated and toxic debris from previous dietary habits. The body's natural cleansing mechanisms are not designed to deal with the unnatural mess that we have created – it requires special methods to eliminate it.

First step: inner cleansing

'By cleaning the gut and bowels we repair not just the mind and the body but also the spirit.'

Cleansing the inner body is an important preliminary step in the path to total health and wellness. Whatever pollutes the body pollutes the mind; whatever pollutes the mind pollutes the spirit, and by cleaning the gut and bowels we repair not just the mind and the body but also the spirit.

Over the years, the number of clients I have seen who have complained about a myriad intestinal conditions has proliferated. They have suffered from general sluggishness, fatigue, brain 'fog', distended abdomen, constipation and bloating, among other symptoms. Others have believed that such symptoms are the 'norm' and have dismissed them as one-off, isolated events.

However, as a professional I know full well that such symptoms are anything but the norm and are often warning signs in the root system of the body: the digestive system and the alimentary canal. Every malfunction of the gut will eventually impact the entire organism, in the same way that a disease in the roots of a tree will have a negative impact on the tree's leaves, its branches and its berries and fruit. If left unchecked, symptoms of malfunction will manifest in the body in the form of a more serious illness. Its cause can often be found everywhere else in the body, rather than the gut.

'The Cleanse made me feel a whole lot better, my eyes are sparkling and I feel "empty". The colonics are a fantastic idea in conjunction with 12 Days ... well recommended.'

Austrian Dr Franz Xaver Mayr, in the twentieth century, asserted the idea that most people's digestive systems were far from clean and were therefore unhealthy. And that even healthy guts contained waste products that caused them to be contaminated, often infected, and therefore were a dangerous source of toxicity. Dr Mayr insisted that anyone who was not completely well should thoroughly cleanse their intestines. He treated all of his patients, regardless of whether they came to him with head, throat, lung, heart or abdominal complaints, as though they had digestive problems. Mayr believed that the toxic gut 'undermined people's health and made them prematurely ill, old, and unattractive.'

The 12-Day Plan, which you will find set out in Part 2 of this book, requires motivation to actively contribute to your healing process and perhaps to give up some long-loved habits – they may be the ones that are the most harmful to you. However, I appreciate that total wellness is not for everybody: amazingly, some people don't actually want to be well. However, you can be as well as you can be. Wellness unfolds gradually through the active participation of the person seeking help, so you owe it to yourself and those around you to be as well as you can be – this is within your ability and power and we all have the ability to improve our own wellness.

Since being well or being sick is mainly rooted in the way that we live and eat, basic good health cannot be 'bought' in a passive way or achieved by simply taking pills – you instead need to fully engage with your own health state. In fact, the better you understand the link between what is allowed, in terms of food and drink, and what is not, and the more you observe the guidelines for carrying out the 12-Day Plan, the more joy, self-confidence and, especially, therapeutic success you will experience in your life.

When practised three or four times a year, particularly if you coincide with the changes in seasons, the 12-Day Plan serves as a remedy and a natural preventative that is fundamentally based on the most ancient remedy to human kind: fasting, purgative herbs and diet.

Fasting and its vital role

'As a medical doctor, I wondered about the rationale of a cleanse. It struck me as simplistic to compare the body to an engine. A simple oil change and everything will be fine. However something profound occurs. Energy and mental clarity are undoubtedly significantly increased. Waking "clear-eyed", so to speak. The 12-day Plan may sound too simple, however simplicity often conceals deep thought and research. To be understood they require a new way of thinking, a change in one's attitude towards self and embracing personal responsibility for our own wellbeing.'

A. SAWYER

'Cleaning up the digestive system is the key to sustainable good health.'

Cleaning up the digestive system is the key to sustainable good health. In the same way that we clean our teeth and wash our hair we should look after our digestive system too. It is part of the parasympathetic nervous system (PNS), which means, like breathing and heartbeat, that it is part of the body that carries on working around the clock. However, as you will see in Part 2, we have a great deal more control than we think we do over the PNS and the gut with the various techniques that are recommended. Many of my clients who come to me with gut issues are prescribed these techniques.

There are no organs or tissues in the body that cannot be damaged by toxins, so it has now been proven that refraining from eating periodically, known as 'intermittent fasting', gives the digestive system time to heal and repair itself, as well as providing other long-term benefits. No method of purging or cleansing is more effective than fasting, which is the treatment par excellence for improving overall health and increasing energy.

Fasting, meaning the temporary, voluntary limitation or complete suspension of food intake, has been known about for thousands of years and practised in many cultures. All of the major religions recommend that its followers cleanse their bodies in order to release them from illness and impurities, and to elevate them to the attainment of higher ends.

Knowledge about fasting was once widespread in the West, particularly in the early schools of philosophy with the Stoics and Epicureans. Even the Greek mathematician and philosopher Pythagoras used to instruct his students to fast before they received his higher teachings. The great physicians of antiquity, such as Hippocrates, often made use of fasting methods too.

How fasting works

Fasting triggers a truly wonderful cleansing process that reaches right down to each and every cell and tissue in the body. Within 24 hours of curtailing eating, enzymes stop entering the stomach and travel instead into the intestines and into the bloodstream, where they circulate and gobble up waste matter, including dead and damaged cells, unwelcome microbes and pollutants. All organs and glands get a much-needed and well-deserved rest, during which time their tissues are purified and rejuvenated and their functions are balanced and regulated. The entire alimentary canal is swept clean and what is eventually eliminated should astonish and disgust first-time fasters in equal measure and encourage them to make fasting and colon-cleansing a life-long habit.

I was personally so impressed with the results of therapeutic fasts when I lived in India that I decided to devote the rest of my life to this method of healing. These experiences encouraged me to develop the 12-Day Plan and make it available for everybody.

My early fasts

When I lived in India, I experimented with many types of fasting. One of my most memorable experiences included living in a cave for ten days with nothing but pure spring water to drink. It was a silent (*mouna*), rent-a-cave arrangement, where my only neighbours were monkeys. A beautiful view stretched before me from the mountaintop cave down to the plains below. In those ten days I explored every area of my psyche. I experienced feelings of gut-wrenching isolation as well as moments of lightness in the form of insane, ecstatic laughter, rounds of self-cuddles, with every psychic state and emotion in between. Days were spent meditating, practising yoga and deep reflection. At the end of ten days I felt lucid, calm, relaxed, un-hungry, detached and self-sufficient. When I was collected afterwards, I was invited for dinner and to share my experience with friends, who had eagerly gathered to hear about it. To my surprise at the time, I declined the invitation, since I just wanted to be alone to process what I had been through.

Today, I always look forward to periods of intermittent fasting (although with a measure of trepidation in the days leading up to it) because it allows me a focused 12-day period of mindfulness that I relish and value highly.

THE DIFFERENCE BETWEEN HUNGER AND FASTING

'Hunger' is a lack of sufficient nutrition to the point where the body suffers, but fasting is the voluntary limitation of food to improve overall health. The entire organism becomes healthy again and there is a positive feeling of harmony between your inner and outer world. When practised over a number of months, intermittent fasting helps to lower blood pressure as well as damaging low-density lipoprotein (LDL) cholesterol, re-balance blood sugar levels and create balance in mind and body.

THE SHANKHAPRAKSHALANA KRIYA TECHNIQUE

When I first started practising yoga in India, Shankhaprakshalana (the kriya technique for cleaning the intestines) was my baptism of fire. This is a practice where the entire alimentary canal is swept clean and what was eliminated astonished and disgusted me in equal measure and made me adopt fasting and colon-cleaning as a life-long habit. What came out very much resembled what you might find on the inside of a car exhaust, and what followed afterwards was a state that could only be likened to a religious experience, a spiritual cleansing or complete paradigm shift of thought. Therefore it's no surprise that cleansing the body is an important preliminary step in certain oriental philosophical systems. Traditionally one of the first-step practices given to a student entering an (continued) ashram in India are cleansing exercises because blocks in the free flow of energy impair health and obstruct the development of higher levels of vitality and awareness.

Having said that, Shankhaprakshalana, or washing of the intestine, should not be undertaken without the assistance of a qualified teacher. It involves having two glasses of warm salt water (two litres in total), followed by dynamic asanas and periodic evacuations, repeated six or seven times. A special meal, usually of khicheri, is eaten about an hour after the practice and then again approximately six hours after this meal, in order to reline the intestines and keep the walls of the gut stretched, otherwise they may cramp. After Shankhaprakshalana, a special diet for at least one month has to be followed as the digestive system becomes temporarily very fragile.

Cleansing the bloodstream

Blood acidosis and inflammation have become a major bane of contemporary civilisation and one of the most important benefits of fasting is that it thoroughly cleanses and purifies the bloodstream. Blood is responsible for delivering nutrients and oxygen to every cell in the body, and it must also carry away metabolic wastes from the cells for excretion in kidney and lungs. Dirty blood simply cannot perform these functions properly. As a result malnutrition sets in, resistance plummets and toxaemia becomes a chronic condition, and germs have a field day invading your most vulnerable tissues.

Fasting re-establishes proper pH balance in the blood.

When acid builds up in the blood, the bloodstream deposits crystals in various joints, where they form 'spurs' that bind your joints together and supplant the synovial fluid that lubricate joints – the result can be painful and lead to debilitating arthritis. However, fasting permits enzymes to enter the joints and dissolve these crystals, thereby restoring the synovial fluids and recovering joint mobility.

Making fasting part of your life

So, unless you live an ascetic life and avoid dietary folly altogether, your blood and other tissues are bound to accumulate toxins and gradually lose their functional vitality. If you do not purge yourself of these toxins on a regular basis, via fasting, toxaemia gets worse, until the body cannot stand it any more, and guess what happens? You get ill.

'The only way to avoid internal and external toxins might be to live an ascetic lifestyle.'

Therefore, if you want to create excellent health in the body and give your gut an occasional rest, I recommend making intermittent fasting part of your normal lifestyle. In any event, it's pointless to embark on a major new dietary plan before you have flushed out all the accumulated and impacted debris from your former dietary habits. There is only one way to do this – and that is by fasting and systematic cleansing and in conjunction with colonic hydrotherapy (if you need it).

The gentle, intermittent fast in my 12-Day Plan takes place during the Power Phase (Days 7–9). This part of the Plan is a liquid-only fast and is manageable and energising, since digestion uses up a lot of energy that can be used elsewhere in the body.

'The first three days were tough. By Day 4 I was feeling good. I've lost seven pounds. I have been having refreshing sleep. I will do the Cleanse again!'

CHAPTER 2

The meaning of stress

S tress is often talked about as being a 'modern' malaise, as though it didn't exist in former times. However, there has always been stress. But these days there always seems to be so much to do in life but not enough time to do it in; what you might call 'the hamster on a wheel syndrome'. The speed of technological advances can help us with gadgets that save us time and, supposedly, stress, but at the same time they compound it. A good example of this is the ability to send and receive emails, texts and phone calls (plus social media communication) wherever you are, so that you never actually relax, switch off and recharge your batteries, away from work and responsibilities.

An antidote to stress and tension is clearly required in our society and one that will be effective in arresting stress-related disorders.

Understanding and managing stress is key to your wellness and your gut is unhappy because of stress. Research has shown that the stress response can alter the natural balance of healthy bacteria in your gut, causing the gut ecosystem to shift in favour of a more hostile group of bacteria. The Mind Body Cleanse techniques described in this book can help and incorporating them as part of your daily routine can take as little as ten minutes every day – however, those few minutes will pay off with great rewards for your gut, stress levels and your general wellness.

Signs of stress

T here are many different symptoms of stress. The body is directly affected by the stress felt in daily life. Here is a list of the commonest signs:

- Muscles tighten and your breath flow decreases.
- Responses to stress are reflected in your posture, which alters according to where and how you hold tension in various parts of your

body – your neck may be bent, causing your head to come forward or your chin juts out, with your whole head moving forward on your neck. Your neck should be lengthened and brought into line with your spine.

■ Stress and tension are also carried in your jaw and face, which appears tight with tension – it should be loose and supple. Your teeth may grind, lips tighten, tongue stick to the roof of your mouth, brows furrow and your eyes screw up.

■ Tension in your shoulders may cause them to lift to your ears or cause them to round. Your shoulders should be wide and relaxed.

■ Your upper arms may stay close to your chest, to your side or in front of your chest.

■ Your elbows may be bent upwards. Your arms should hang easily from wide and relaxed shoulders.

■ Your chest tends to be caved in and constricted, whereas it needs to be opened out and widened.

■ Your fingers and thumbs curl to make a fist or your hands may clench each other. There should be space between your fingers – not too much space so that tension is created, but not too little so that your fingers remain inactive.

■ Your spine may be rigid and locked – it needs to be relaxed and extended upwards.

■ Tension in your pelvis causes it to be locked back. It needs to drop forwards slightly, under your upper body. Tucking the tailbone under helps.

■ Your legs may be stiff with tension; they should be loose and flexible. Both men and women tend to show tension by crossing their legs, holding the top foot rigid, or moving the ankle up and down. While standing, you may tend to cross and uncross your legs and walk about distractedly.

■ Your knees may be stiff and locked, whereas they should be loose and flexible.

■ You may hold your upper body rigid and lean forward, which will eventually cause pain in your back. Your feet should be stable and shoulder-width apart in order to support your body weight evenly.

While some stress is inevitable in our lives, such as the positive stress created in order to be able to get up and dressed in the morning, too much stress can lead to harmful emotional and physical side effects.

Physical indications of stress may include:

- Repeated headaches
- Heart palpitations
- Chest pain and tightness
- Sweating
- Indigestion
- Breathlessness
- Nausea
- Muscle twitches
- Tiredness
- Dizziness
- Vague aches or pains
- Skin irritation or rashes
- Susceptibility to allergies
- Fainting
- Frequent colds
- Flu or other infections
- Recurrence of previous illnesses
- Constipation or diarrhoea
- Rapid weight gain or loss
- Alteration of the menstrual pattern (in women).

The emotional signs of stress may include:

- Mood swings
- Increased worrying
- Irritability
- Feeling tense
- Feeling drained
- Lack of enthusiasm
- Feeling cynical
- Feeling a sense of rising panic
- Apprehension
- Feelings helpless
- Loss of confidence
- Lack of self-esteem
- Lack of concentration
- Withdrawal into daydreaming

- Overreacting to things unnecessarily or unrelated to the cause of the stress
- Overactive imagination or fast and negative internal dialogue
- Being short-tempered and snappy with others.

The psychological signs of stress may include:
- Not having clearly defined goals
- Being uncertain about the future
- Feeling powerless to change or influence your individual circumstances
- Believing that your opinion doesn't matter, isn't heard or valued
- Feeling judged, criticised or ignored by others
- Bullying or unreasonable behaviour – a manifestation of insecurity
- Believing that working hard or being successful is the key to being a 'good' person
- Having regrets about the past and what could have been
- Feeling stuck in relationships or jobs that aren't working but being afraid to make changes
- Not having the skills or the confidence to carry out a task and feeling that admitting this would be a sign of weakness
- Living a life/doing a job or career that you fell into or someone else chose for you, but which isn't actually what you really want to do in life.

The behavioural signs of stress may include:
- Lack of energy
- Accident-proneness
- Poor standards of work
- Increased smoking
- Increased consumption of alcohol
- Increased dependence on drugs
- Overeating or loss of appetite
- Change in sleep patterns
- Difficulty in getting to sleep and waking up tired
- Loss of interest in sex
- Poor time management
- Impaired speech
- Withdrawal from supportive relationships

- Taking work home more
- Being too busy to relax
- Generally not looking after oneself.

Tips to help you manage stress:
- Anticipate stressful periods and plan for them
- Know your individual warning signs and stress triggers and catch them early
- Develop a number of constructive strategies and practise them (get enough sleep, eat a balanced diet to maintain correct weight and do enjoyable exercise)
- Smoke and drink alcohol and caffeine in moderation, or not at all
- Avoid eating refined and processed foods
- Do not suppress your feelings; acknowledge them to yourself and share them with someone you trust
- Learn to be more flexible and adaptable
- Avoid blaming others for situations
- Provide positive feedback to others
- Learn to say no and be more assertive
- Be receptive when genuine help is offered
- Use free time productively (pamper yourself in a way that is right for you: massage, listen to music, have a hot bath, watch a comedy show, etc.)
- Take 30 minutes each day to take stock and refine how and when to deal with the causes of stress
- Book a specific appointment after your normal working day (e.g. an evening class once a week – so that you have to leave work on time)
- Take mini breaks during the day and stretch your limbs
- Increase your self-awareness and knowledge by reading 'self-help' books
- Plan ahead for weekends away and holidays to wind down and de-stress
- Attend a stress-management course or read stress-management books
- Seek out variety and change of pace in your life
- Spend time in nature and enjoy simple, enjoyable things (e.g. kicking autumn leaves)

- Remember to attend to your spiritual development
- Maintain a sense of proportion at all times.

Mastering discomfort

When people are stressed, they often turn to cigarettes, alcohol, drugs, gambling, shopping, food – anything to 'get rid' of their feelings of discomfort or feelings they don't like. However, if you take a deeper look at the stress, it's probably an unfounded fear that's causing it (this is usually the fear that we're not good enough), and if we examine that fear and give it the light of day, it will start to go away, to melt and disappear.

'If you take a deeper look at the stress, it's really an unfounded fear that's causing it.'

By the time stress has manifested in the body it is too late – it has become symptomatic. This is the precise moment that people come to one of my Mind Body Cleanse classes or workshops, expecting that the postures and breathing practices I teach them will deal with their stress – not a bad guess, in fact. However, the truth is that we can do all of the neck rolls, Downward-facing Dogs, shoulder balances to help to relieve tension in the musculature of the upper body, where stress collects, but it is far better to deal with the root cause of stress rather than waiting for it to become symptomatic.

Don't be a comfort addict

Of all the skills I have learned since I first started on my spiritual journey in India many years ago, a particular one stands out, and that is: learning to be comfortable with discomfort – and that includes the discomfort of stress.

If you learn this skill, you can master pretty much anything that life throws at you. It might sound counter-intuitive, but discomfort can be the joyful key that opens up everything for you. You can climb a mountain, beat your tendency for procrastination, make your diet healthier, explore new things, speak on stage, start exercising, learn a new language, eradicate clutter in your home, make it through tough times, write a book – all of these things can be sources of stress.

Unfortunately, most people avoid discomfort. I mean – they *really* avoid it. At the first sign of discomfort, they'll run as fast as they can in the other direction; spend money, take pills, eat unhealthy foods or indulge in some other form of toxic therapy. These people mistakenly believe that their discomfort will go away as a result; I call these people 'comfort addicts'.

Comfort addicts are the types of people who don't eat vegetables because they think they don't 'like' the taste (or they disliked it when they were children, their parents failed to address the issue and they never grew out of it). And so they eat what they have already grown to like since childhood, which may well turn out to be sweets, fried foods, meats, cheeses, salty things and lots of processed flour goods. These people don't like things that feel uncomfortable, but in the long run they will create a life that is deeply uncomfortable as a result because their health will deteriorate.

The wonderful thing I have learned in my own practice is that a little discomfort isn't actually a bad thing. In fact, with a little training, discomfort can be something you can enjoy. When I discovered this, I was able to change everything and even start enjoying my yoga practice! Now a little discomfort has become part of my master plan.

CHAPTER 3

The vital role of the gut

How the digestive system works

To fully understand the central importance of the role of the gut in your health and wellness, and how it is of key importance to the Mind Body Cleanse ethos, we must first explore how it works. Then, in Part 2, we show you how the 12-Day Plan can help you if you are struggling with sluggish intestines and other gut-related conditions.

'The intestines are the Father of all suffering.'

OLD ARABIC SAYING

The strength of a tree does not lie in its limbs or branches, but in its roots. And the root system of the human body is not found in the hand or in the feet, but in the digestive organs. Like the roots of a tree, the digestive organs process food, extract vital nutrients and deliver them to the rest of the organism. They also excrete the rubbish generated by metabolism.

The digestive system is a tube-shaped canal, which is up to 27 feet long in adults. The surface area of the gut is 200 times greater than the skin, making it the largest surface of interaction with the world. It begins at the mouth and ends at the anus and includes the oesophagus, stomach, and small and large intestines. The liver, the gall bladder, the pancreas, as well as billions of mucus glands in the stomach and intestines, are each a part of it. Just as the roots of a plant absorb nourishment from the earth, producing branches, leaves and blossoms, millions of intestinal villi take root in the chyme, absorbing food that has broken down in the gut and supply it to the bloodstream, which in turn carries it to the 60 trillion cells of the human body.

How the digestive system works
The mouth

Digestion begins in the mouth with the production of ptyalin, a digestive enzyme secreted at the very first sight, smell or even thought of food.

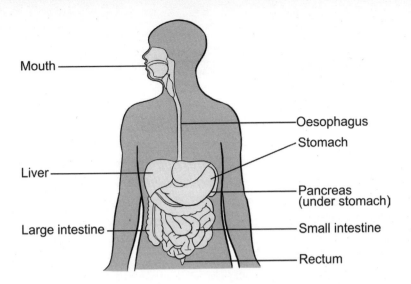

Mouth

Oesophagus

Stomach

Liver

Pancreas
(under stomach)

Large intestine

Small intestine

Rectum

Masticating your food thoroughly is key to good digestion and food should enter the stomach as a thick liquid, not hastily swallowed, unchewed chunks or lumps. The papillae in your cheeks and beneath your tongue secrete around 0.7 litres of saliva every day, which starts off the digestive process.

If you explore the root of the tongue with your finger, you will notice bumpy nodules. This area, known as the lingual tonsils, contains immune tissue. The job of these nodules is to analyse tiny particles of everything that you eat. Before we reach about seven years of age, our tonsils are still an important training camp for our immune cells. Building a strong immune system is key to keeping the heart healthy and in controlling body weight. It is worth noting that removing the tonsils of a child younger than age seven can lead to an increased risk of obesity.

The oesophagus

On the arrival of the bolus of food, the oesophagus choreographs a wave-like action to draw the food downwards towards the stomach. This propulsive peristalsis is so much a part of our physiology that it even works if you are standing on your head. In this first part of the digestive journey, the conscious peripheral nervous system and the autonomic nervous system – or that part of the nervous system that we can influence – work in harmony.

The stomach

The position of the stomach is much higher in the upper body than we realise. It begins at the left nipple and ends below the bottom of the ribcage, on the right-hand side, behaving a bit like a washing machine, slapping and turning, churning and walloping food against its back wall to ensure that it can be absorbed in the small and large intestines. From here, food particles are ground into tiny particles that then pass into the small intestine.

Liquid travels down the shorter right-hand side of the stomach to end up at the entrance to the small intestine. Food, on the other hand, travels against the larger side of the stomach and gets smashed to the sides.

Immediately before food arrives in the stomach, the latter relaxes so that it can stretch and extend for as long as it needs to. Emotions such as anxiety or fear inhibit the stomach from relaxing, which can stop us feeling hungry or make us feel nauseous. If you have difficulty winding down and relaxing before eating, I recommend a few different short breathing practices before eating, which influence the rest and relaxation response. These simple practices ensure that everything in the stomach is working in the way that it should before you eat (see Three-part breath and complete breath, page 115).

Stress not only affects your mental state but can also take its toll on your physical wellbeing. It can negatively affect every part of your digestive system, causing your gut, and especially your colon, to spasm or even increase the acid in your stomach, causing indigestion.

The pH of the stomach is very acidic and activates peptidases that begin to break down proteins. While simple carbohydrates, such as pasta or rice, pass into the small intestine quite quickly, proteins and fats need a great deal more work to process them, which requires greater energy. This is why I recommend not eating animal protein during the 12-Day Plan. A piece of steak, for example, may easily be churned around in the stomach for between five and seven hours and therefore consumes too much energy.

The acidic environment of the stomach is also a first line of defence against harmful bacteria in our food. In the stomach, carbohydrates break down into glucose. Protein is broken down into amino acids, the building blocks of muscle and tissue.

The small intestine
Ninety per cent of all foodstuffs are absorbed through the wall of the small intestine, where bacteria that naturally live in our gut begin fermenting and feeding off our food. The small intestine is between 3 and 6 metres long. As food moves into the small intestine, the pH changes from being acidic to more alkaline. The small intestine absorbs, through billions of finger-like projections called villi, the nutrients derived from the combination of mono-saccharide carbohydrates, which come from vegetables and fruits are easy to digest – with proteins from animal sources and essential fats found in fish, nuts and seeds. In the final stages of food breakdown in the small intestine, our digestive enzymes work like tiny scissors and break down food to the same basic ingredients: sugar molecules, amino acids and fats. The villi help to move the chyme down the digestive line, where everything is moving forwards. The action of peristalsis is greatly enhanced by Mind Body Cleanse twisting movements, which you will find in Part 2 (see pages 130–3, 146–51 and 182). These yogic twisting poses bring intelligence into the gut and the action of pushing and pulling with the breath in turn speeds metabolism and digestion.

The large intestine
The health of the large intestine is dependent on the smooth functioning of all the digestive functions in harmony.

The large intestine is the home of our gut flora, dealing with anything that gets swept into the large intestine undigested, and it needs time to complete this action. Water is absorbed and any remaining nutrients, including energy-rich fatty acids, vitamin K, vitamin B12, B1 and B2. The colon takes its time with all the leftovers and digests them thoroughly. During this time it processes calcium, which can only be absorbed properly in the colon. Everything is then screened by the liver before entering the main blood system.

The large intestine, unlike other parts of the gut, also has to deal with the brain directly: it is the brain that decides when it wants to make the colon evacuate its contents, not the large intestine. Sometimes, when we are anxious, the brain orders the large intestine into evacuation, without sufficient time to reabsorb all the water the body lent it. The result is diarrhoea. This is why engaging with the parasympathetic branch of the autonomic nervous system (R&R response) before eating as described in Part 2 (see three-part breath and complete breath, page 115) is key if you are prone to runny tummies.

On average, food movement from fork to toilet can take one day, while those who provide the intestine with sufficient bulk may have to go to the toilet two or three times a day. Slower guts can take as many as three to four days for the food to pass through. Generally speaking, women's large intestines are slightly slower than men's.

ARE YOU SITTING COMFORTABLY?

Even in our modern world, most people, globally, still defecate in the squatting position – especially in Asia, the Middle East and Africa. It is only in the industrialised West, where the modern toilet, or 'throne', was invented, that people sit on something in order to defecate, using the same posture as when they sit down on a chair to eat.

Anatomically speaking, the 'throne' is a device of considerable torture to the bowels. When sitting on a 'throne', the lower end of the descending colon is bent, requiring a major muscular effort to evacuate the bowels. The intense effort required can lead to clogging the minute capillaries that feed the anal sphincter, and this may lead to the formation of haemorrhoids and bleeding piles.

When squatting, however, the colon naturally aligns itself with the rectum and anus, and no, or very little, effort is required for evacuation. In fact, you will evacuate so much more in a single, efficient squatting than you will in a single sitting. No wonder so many in the Western world suffer from chronic constipation!

In southern India, nearly 20 years ago, I was in a place called Patnem. I rented a beach hut and on the first night I was given a pig. I couldn't quite work out what this pig was for until the following morning, when I went to perform my ablutions. There are no Western-style toilets in that part of India, and I had become quite used to squatting to eliminate waste. It had even begun to feel quite comfortable – until I saw the pig's snout and two eyes peering up at me expectedly through the hole in the toilet bowl!

LET'S GET THINGS MOVING

Increasing fibre
Unless you are attempting to target a specific health goal, such as lowering your cholesterol, which requires more soluble fibre, in general focus on eating foods that span the colours of the rainbow. This way you will be getting all the soluble and insoluble fibres required for a healthy diet in the phytonutrient spectrum. The best way to increase your fibre intake is to *gradually* incorporate more foods in this list (see page 58). If you are increasing the intake of fibre in your diet, make sure you increase your water intake too. Not drinking enough water when increasing fibre intake can lead to constipation.

The issue of constipation
The best barometer for assessing constipation is not how often you need to go to the toilet, but how difficult it is. Temporary constipation can be due to stress, travelling or illness. Prolonged symptoms can point to more serious conditions.

You can try the following to get things moving:
> Take psyllium husks and/or prune fibre. Both contain fibre and also draw extra fluids into the gut. Be patient – it can take three days to take effect.
> Drink more fluids – this may be very helpful. Air travel can cause the body to lose water, without even sweating, so it's vital to drink plenty of water before, during and after flights.
> Try not to put yourself under pressure to go to the loo; your gut likes to work according to plan so if you need to go, just go!

The most common effect of sluggish bowels is the formation of toxins from decomposition. Just as butter goes rancid and fruit begins to ferment, and while meat goes bad, likewise a sluggish intestine forms poisons. This may lead to gastritis and gastroptosis, intestinal ulcers and various diseases of the intestines. Fasting and cleansing should be done as a preventative measure.

The pancreas
The pancreas secretes pancreatic juice, which is alkaline, to neutralise the acid from the stomach. It performs two major tasks. It produces:
- Enzymes (for digestion); protease (for proteins); amylase (for carbohydrates); and lipase (for fats) to aid digestion in the small intestine
- Hormones: insulin to help regulate blood-sugar levels by transporting glucose to the brain and muscles for energy, and leptin to tell your brain when you are full.

The liver
In the liver, bile salts serve to emulsify fats from the food we eat. Eating the right kind of fat feeds the body with nutrient-dense compounds that are vital for the brain and nervous system and helps to produce hormones. The liver is also the primary organ of detoxification, processing all toxins that we absorb from the environment.

COLONIC HYDROTHERAPY

Colonic irrigation cleanses the entire colon from the ascending portion across the transverse portion to the descending portion of the colon. The procedure must not be confused with enemas (at best, enemas flush out the rectum and a small part of the descending colon, but they do not reach the transverse and ascending portions).

Colonic hydrotherapy should work entirely by gravity rather than via pumping and it is vital that it is administered by a professional. You can use ARCH, which is registered in the UK and Europe.

Russian physicians realise that no cure for any ailment can be properly administered to an 'unclean', highly toxic, body, which simply cannot assimilate medication.

So in Russia it remains standard procedure in all hospitals and clinics to administer a thorough colonic cleansing to all patients, regardless of their ailments, immediately upon arrival.

The roles of the gut

The multiple functions of the gut interact with each other and with the food you eat to regulate your nutrition, metabolism, mental function, weight, energy and your susceptibility to illness.

- Your gut has its own nervous system, the enteric nervous system (ENS), which has as many nerve cells as your spinal column and has constant contact with your brain. This has a direct impact on your mood and mental function.
- Your gut is also home to about 100 trillion microbes and lives in a symbiotic relationship with favourable bacteria, yeast and fungi, viruses and an occasional worm. This is called the 'microbiome'.
- Over two-thirds of your body's immune system is found in the lining of the small intestine. Thus your gut is the largest immune barrier to the outside world.
- The gut is also an organ of detoxification. Much of this responsibility rests with the liver, but the intestinal lining cells are themselves rich in detoxifying enzymes.

The mind gut

'The state of your guts affects how you feel in your mind.'

The state of your guts affects how you feel in your mind. It can be either a source of suffering or of extraordinary wellness. The gut is home to an unimaginable number of nerves and it commands fleets of signalling substances and connections.

Just as the brain has its own nervous system, the central nervous system (CNS), the gut has its own nervous system called the enteric nervous system (ENS). Both systems originate from the same embryonic tissues and in life share a certain synchronicity.

The ENS has a number of key functions. It:
- Controls the immune system in the gut
- Coordinates the release of hormones as food arrives
- Helps to open up the gut to circulation after you eat, which help absorption of nutrients
- Choreographs and coordinates the contraction of the muscle cells that line the intestines to keep everything moving in the right direction (i.e. out of the body).

The ENS is autonomous. If the connection between the enteric nervous system and the brain is severed at the vagus nerve, the gut will continue to function as if nothing has happened. It will even continue to digest food! This is unique to the ENS and is found nowhere else in the body.

The gut is affectionately referred to as the 'second brain' and the conversation that takes place between the first brain and the second brain is actually a two-way-highway conversation, although it has to be said that 90 per cent of the conversation is from the gut to the brain.

The vagus nerve

The insular cortex part of the brain needs information from the vagus to form a picture of how the body is doing. So, while the vagus nerve works like a telephone cable between the switchboard, or brain, the ENS gathers information from the gut. This makes the gut the largest sensory organ to the outside world. The information that the ENS gathers is used by the conscious mind.

A healthy gut does not transmit unimportant signals from the gut to the brain via the vagus nerve. However, if the gut thinks that something is important, it may require the brain's input rather than process it with its own brain.

Listening to your gut

The gut is not only the seat of your health, it is also the seat of your intuition; a huge matrix that senses our inner life working on the subconscious mind.

Human beings have an innate ability to process information about what's going on around them and put a response into action separate from the brain and the central nervous system.

Listening to your gut is a very visceral activity; it is like having a sixth sense. In fact, listening to gut feelings is the most powerful guiding ally we have – ignoring them often leads to suffering. Cooperation between the gut and brain begins very early in life. When we are children we have not yet evolved the analytical brain to override what we are truly feeling and are adept at responding to the impulses from the gut, but as we get older we experience the world more through our senses.

BUTTERFLY FEELINGS

Have you ever felt 'butterflies' in your tummy? Underlying this sensation is an often-overlooked network of neurons lining the gut.

You don't have to be a gastroenterologist to be aware of the more subtle feelings in your stomach that accompany emotions such as excitement, fear and stress. The second brain consists of sheaths of neurons embedded in the walls of the long tube of our gut, or alimentary canal. The second brain contains some 100 million neurons, more than in either the spinal cord or the peripheral nervous system. It is this multitude of neurons in the enteric nervous system that enables us to 'feel' the inner world of our gut.

'Listening to your gut is a very visceral response; it is like having a sixth sense.'

You can become more sensitive to the mind – gut connection. The Mind Body Cleanse techniques that we look at in Part 2 will help you to explore and strengthen this vital connection.

As adults we have to practise letting go of the analytical and over-thinking mind and trust in our intuition, especially when it comes to assessing potentially threatening situations. The process of making decisions based on gut feeling may involve the gut recalling how it felt in similar situations in the past. This is why yoga and meditation are such good, effective practices – because they allow us to step back, drop the analytical mind and tune in to our intuition. Therefore developing our intuition, with the help of techniques described in the second half of this book, allows us to have more control over our own health.

The microbiome

I was recently delivering a presentation on Mind Body Cleanse techniques, in leafy south-west London. A top fashion designer was in the audience and needed encouragement to sit still. I said to the lady: 'You are 90 per cent bacteria, and 10 per cent human.' As you would imagine, this did not go down too well. Most people do not like to think of themselves as consisting mostly of bacteria, and for this reason the fashion designer looked aghast, but at last started to pay attention to the presentation!

'You are 90 per cent bacteria, and 10 per cent human.'

Viewed at great magnification, bacteria resemble bright little spots against a black background. The microbiome and its role in maintaining health and healing disease is one of the greatest medical discoveries in modern science. It comprises all the microorganisms inhabiting us.

There is an inconceivable number of microbes in the gut and, according to recent research, humans are made up primarily of bacterial cells that control virtually every aspect of our physiology. It is vital to our wellness that we shatter the myth that bacteria are the 'enemy'. The bacteria of the microbiome are actually our greatest allies when it comes to improving health.

If you lifted out your gut, you would find that your microbiome weighed up to two kilos and contain about 100 trillion bacteria. One gram of faeces contains more bacteria than there are people on earth.

Some scientists now support the theory that our gut microbiota can be considered an organ in its own right. It has an origin, develops with us, is made up of trillions of cells, and is in constant contact with its fellow organs.

Bacteria help to:
- Break down foodstuffs
- Supply the gut with energy
- Manufacture vitamins
- Train our immune system.

The precise nature of the creatures that colonise us makes a difference to our wellbeing. Varying proportions of different bacteria in our gut have been detected in those suffering from obesity, nervous disorders, depression and even malnutrition. So, when something is wrong with our microbiome, something is wrong with us!

Science is just beginning to understand that we are all individual ecosystems:

- The numbers of bacteria are greater in the colon and rectum, rather than higher up in the gut.
- Bacteria do not like to be removed from their own world and it is very difficult to observe them.
- Our gastrointestinal tract is home to more than a thousand species of bacteria – plus populations of viruses and yeasts and fungi.
- If we allow the wrong bacteria to colonise our gut, which produces a variety of different toxins, we may end up with all sorts of behavioural and emotional problems. Our brain chemistry can be changed for the worse.
- If you add this deteriorating condition to the immune response, which includes the effects of inflammation, this can affect the brain too, with the result that your central nervous system becomes inflamed.

The brain cannot work effectively unless it is working in an environment that is anti-inflammatory. And to work on the brain you have to start with the gut.

The development of gut flora

The moment each of us passes through the birth canal, a unique combination of microbes from our mother's vagina initiates the process of colonising our bodies, both inside our airways and digestive tract, and outside on our skin. Up until this point we live in an environment that is germ-free inside our mother's womb. At the age of three our gut flora develops to the right level and then stabilises, after our bacterium has gone through the wars, so to speak. And so begins the long process of bacterial colonisation, the composition of which depends upon our own actions – largely due to what we put in our mouths!

One-third of all children in the Western, industrialised, world are born via Caesarean section. And these children, including myself, have to garner bacteria from somewhere, since their population will not develop from the mother's vagina. Children born by Caesarean section take much longer to develop a normal population of gut bacteria. They also have an increased risk of developing allergies or asthma.

Breastfeeding promotes specific members of our gut microbiotica, such as bifidobacteria. These bacteria are integral to the development of the immune system in later life. Interestingly, children with insufficient bifidobacteria have an increased risk of developing obesity in later life.

While our genes help to design our bodies, they do not design our microbial home. Taken together, our gut bacteria have 150 times more genes than a human being. This massive collection of genes is called a 'biome'. And their genes represent a huge pool of borrowed abilities.

Our bacterial colonies change with lifestyle, diet and our exposure to antibiotics. This microbiome of 100 trillion tiny creatures dictates how our bodies feel, how our immune systems behave, and how we digest foods. However, we are only at the beginning of learning how the bacteria of the gut can have an effect on an adult human.

How might gut bacteria make us fat?

The idea that the bacteria in our gut might influence our overall metabolism, and therefore our weight, is only a recent phenomenon. A hypothesis postulated in 2013 suggests that gut bacteria can affect the appetite of the host. It is our bacteria that reward us when we send them a decent delivery of food. They do this by cranking up the body's production of certain transmitters. This principle applies to the feeling of satiety.

When we consider the range of functions carried out by our microbiome, it is not surprising that these microbes are able to express their wishes too. We do, after all, live symbiotically with our bacteria.

The nutrition we receive from bacteria is not only important for fighting flab, it also affects the levels of fats, such as cholesterol, in our blood.

Obesity and high cholesterol are connected with the greatest health issues of our time: hypertension, arteriosclerosis and diabetes.

CHOLESTEROL-LOWERING BACTERIA?

The early indications are that the bacterium *Lactobacillus plantarum* can significantly lower high cholesterol and other blood lipid levels, increase 'good' HDL cholesterol and lead to significantly lower rates of arteriosclerosis.

Follow-up research still needs to be carried out to verify these promising indications. *Lactobacillus plantarum* is already recommended as a pain treatment for patients with IBS.

Our bacteria do not take anything from us when they share food. Remember that 90 per cent of our digestion takes place in the small intestine, where we absorb most of our nutrients, whereas the highest concentration of bacteria is found where digestion has nearly finished. If this equilibrium is disturbed and bacteria migrate to the small intestine, we may come across what doctors call 'bacterial overgrowth'. This can cause severe bloating, abdominal pain, joint pain, nutrient deficiencies and anaemia.

Bacteria do more than just break down food. They also produce completely new substances. Fresh cabbage, for example, is less rich in vitamins than the sauerkraut it can be turned into. Extra vitamins are made by our bacteria.

'With the right amount of healthy bacteria, our guts can promote happy brains.'

Unfortunately, over the years our modern diet, full of sugar, processed foods and additives, promotes the growth of harmful bacteria and yeast. It also turns on genes that are unfavourable to our wellbeing. With the right amount of healthy bacteria, our guts can promote happy minds. However, if the wrong yeast and bacteria start to colonise the gut, toxins are produced which in the long run can create problems.

Your gut and your brain will function optimally when their signals are not jammed by toxins, food allergens and stress. I am always amazed at how lucid my thinking becomes after completing the 12-Day Plan. My problem-solving skills are also greatly improved.

The immune system and our bacteria

Several times a day our lives are saved by our immune system. Mutated cells are destroyed, bacteria are peppered with holes and viruses are sliced in two. The immune system has to tread delicately in the gut; while it permits peaceful co-existence with the many bacteria that live there, it must also be able to recognise enemies. Our immune system must also be able to differentiate between its own cells and the body's own human cells. It doesn't always. Type 1 diabetes results from the autoimmune destruction of the cells that produce insulin.

The gut is the training camp for the immune system. And immune cells with a tendency to attack the body's own tissue are weeded out before they leave the camp.

When it comes to the immune system, much of what bacteria tends to do is 'fine-tuning'. Each kind of bacterium has its own way of affecting the immune system. Some species of bacteria have been observed to make our immune system more tolerant by producing mediatory immune cells, while others have been found to provoke the immune system by imitating the behaviour of more harmful pathogens. For example, these provocateurs might dock in the villi of the small intestine. When a dangerous pathogen passes by, the provocateur has already docked in their favourite spot and it will move on. This phenomenon is known as 'colonisation resistance'. The majority of the microbes in our gut protect us simply by occupying spaces that would otherwise be free for harmful bacteria to colonise.

Antibiotics – against life

Antibiotics kill bacteria by filling them with holes, by poisoning bacteria, or by destroying bacteria's ability to reproduce. However, antibiotics are oversubscribed and often prescribed as if they were ordinary sweets from a sweetshop – this is a huge problem. Antibiotics decimate the microbiome and this can eventually lead to serious health problems.

The main reason for taking antibiotics is to cure 'colds'. However, as any family doctor will tell you, most infections are viral, whereas antibiotics only kill bacteria. Except for a select few, viruses are unaffected by antibiotics. Most colds are caused by viruses and will resolve with some simple rest and immune support. So, taking antibiotics for a cold is a complete waste of time and will negatively affect your delicate microbiome.

When medically necessary, for example in cases of severe pneumonia, or for helping children recover from an acute infection, taking antibiotics can be justified. The cost is high in terms of the price you pay for the destruction of good bacteria in your gut, which could take many years to recover, but overall, in this situation, the risk is worth taking.

Antibiotics can alter gut flora. Our microbe collection becomes less diverse and their ability to produce vitamins is affected, likewise the amount of cholesterol they can absorb and the type of foodstuffs they can help us digest. Most of all, antibiotics can be a problem for old people and children.

However, the over-subscription of antibiotics is leading to more antibiotic-resistant bacteria that are difficult to treat and can kill. Many thousands of people die in the West because they are infected with bacteria that have developed resistances that no drug can counter. And every time you take a course of antibiotics your gut flora is changed.

After a course of antibiotics it is essential to repopulate the gut with good bacteria. This can be achieved through eating fermented foods or by taking a multi-strain probiotic. If you do not take care of yourself after a course of antibiotics, you can suffer from an imbalance between good bacteria and bad bacteria, as your gut flora changes.

HOW TO KEEP OUT OF THE ANTIBIOTIC WARS

> Do not take antibiotics unless it is 100 per cent necessary to do so
> Always complete your course of antibiotics
> Buy organically farmed meat
> Wash your fruit and vegetables

> Take care when travelling and follow this advice: 'If you can't peel it, cook it or boil it, don't touch it!'

Yeast, the gut and the brain

The overuse of antibiotics is the root cause for the overgrowth of yeast in the gut. Eating high-sugar foods feeds the yeast and creates neurotoxins, which are responsible for fatigue, mental fog, mood swings, poor memory, insomnia, anxiety, muscle and joint pains and depression. Accompanying the yeast overgrowth is usually a 'leaky' gut. The yeast passes through the cheesecloth-like gut lining, causing all sorts of problems such as body pain and fibromyalgia. Many students have come to me over the years complaining of doctors who are unable to resolve their issues and they have asked me if yoga can help soothe their painful muscles. And after a few months of practice, which often includes the 12-Day Plan, their symptoms start to slowly dissipate.

Dysbiosis

Dysbiosis is a microbial imbalance inside the gut, characterised by increased levels of harmful bacteria, yeast and parasites, and reduced levels of beneficial bacteria.

Between the antibiotics, poor dietary habits and the toxins that you are exposed to in your environment, and the resulting dysbiosis, you put yourself at risk to processes in the body such as a leaky gut.

Other common causes of dysbiosis include:
- Chronic indigestion
- Constipation
- Stress.

The symptoms of dysbiosis are non-specific and can be seen if you suffer from the following:
- Gas
- Bloating
- Indigestion
- Constipation.

Symptoms outside your gut include:
- Asthma
- Eczema
- Rashes

- Nerve pain
- Joint swelling.

Candida/yeast overgrowth

Yeast overgrowth is a form of yeast dysbiosis. Your best protection against this is a normal acidic stomach pH, but any acid-blocking medication may lead to yeast overgrowth. If yeast overgrowth establishes itself, toxins produced by it will create problems in the body and may lead to further conditions, which may seem unrelated at first. A diet rich in sugar and simple carbohydrates is usually the culprit.

Common symptoms of yeast overgrowth:
- Fatigue
- Mental fog
- Anxiety
- Joint pains
- Itchiness
- Bloating.

Probiotics and prebiotics

As we have seen, every time you take antibiotics your gut flora is disrupted. That's trillions (more than there are stars in the Milky Way) of microbes, whose delicate balance influences our overall health. A disruption here allows pathogenic bacteria to step in and it can take over. Probiotics help the gut to return to a state of healthy equilibrium.

People have been taking probiotics since ancient times; our ancestors used bacteria to preserve food. Every culture in the world uses microbes in food preparation. Germany has its sauerkraut, the French have their crème fraîche and the Turks have their ayran. And in Asian cultures we have miso soup, lassi, etc. All these foods rely on fermentation.

Friendly bacteria help us to maintain proper intestinal permeability. They help to stabilise the villi in the gut, which is likely to grow bigger because of their presence. The more stable they are the less waste they will allow through the gut wall.

One of their most important jobs is to defend the gut, and outnumber and antagonise unwelcome pathogens in it. These unwelcome pathogens could be parasites, yeast or bacteria. This activity known as 'colonisation resistance' prevents colonisation of our guts by unfavourable pathogens.

Probiotics are really our silent heroes of health and have been shown to decrease the frequency of sinus, ear and upper-respiratory infections in children. And not only do they protect us against pathogens but they also help to reduce 'leakiness' of the gut and bolster our immune system as well.

A number of fermented foods can support the growth and proliferation of your 'good' bacteria.

Try to incorporate:
- Cultured foods, such as yoghurts and kefir
- Fermented foods
- Coconut water kefir.

However, when completing the 12-Day Plan, it is best to avoid dairy foods for 12 days.

Probiotics for life

Normally probiotics require refrigeration. There are several supplements on the market; however, I find the best ones to use are those that have at least 16 viable strains that have been subjected to rigorous scientific study and are proven to be effective. Strain-level research is key, and you can be sure that the strains are of the highest quality and backed by solid scientific research. I selected 16 key strains in my product 'Brilliant Biotic' (see page 202) because science has demonstrated that to be an optimum amount for the vast majority of people to attain and maintain a healthy gut. The sicker your gut is, the more imbalanced it is, the higher the dose will be needed to create a positive effect. Brilliant Biotic can also guarantee 30 billion live microorganisms at the time of expiration, rather than just at the time of manufacture. See page 202 for a list of the active ingredients included in Brilliant Biotic.

Take Brilliant Biotic on an empty stomach at least twice a day for at least three months to:

- Regulate local and systemic immune function
- Regulate inflammation
- Regulate bowel motility
- Support mucosal barrier
- Support resistance to pathogens.

Lactobacillus and bifidobacterium   Some of the most beneficial Lactobacillus probiotics are *L. acidophilus, L. plantarum* and *L. paracasei*. They help to repopulate the small intestine with friendly organisms that will help support digestion and the performance of the immune system.

Bifidobacteria (Bifidus) predominantly live in the colon or large intestine. *Bifidobacteria lactis* helps support intestinal motility, promotes immune balance and relieves IBS symptoms. They produce butyrate, which is essential for the health of the cells that line the colon.

Prebiotics – before life

Whereas probiotics are live microorganisms and are responsible for boosting your digestion and reducing bad levels of 'bad' gut bacteria and strengthening the immune system, prebiotics are non-digestible ingredients that pass undigested into the large intestine, where they feed our beneficial bacteria. Nothing influences our gut as much as the food we eat. And we should feed our microbes well so they can populate as much of the large intestine as possible. We need to include real roughage, made of real fibre in fruit and vegetables.

Prebiotics can:

- Influence the composition of the gut microbiome
- Prevent infections
- Regulate appetite
- Prevent neoplastic changes
- Increase nutrient utilisation.

The best way to take prebiotics   is to eat them. But introduce them slowly into your diet, otherwise things can get a little gassy.

Top foods containing prebiotics (all raw):

- Chicory root
- Jerusalem artichoke
- Dandelion greens
- Garlic
- Leeks
- Onions
- Asparagus
- Banana (not during the 12-Day Plan).

Prebiotics support our good gut bacteria by eating certain foods. This results in a reduction of toxins produced in the gut. In fact, prebiotics are much more suitable for daily use than probiotics. And they only require one condition: beneficial bacteria must already be present in the gut.

Why probiotics help you lose belly fat

If your gut is not as healthy as it could be, your stomach will always be fat. Probiotics help you to lose weight around your stomach because they help ensure that your digestive system is working to the best of its ability. They also help your body absorb health-boosting nutrients from your food better.

'Mental illnesses' of the gut

For hundreds of years, people have believed that the gut interacts with the brain to influence health and disease. However, the brain also interacts with, and affects, the gut. Depression treatments that target the mind can unintentionally impact the gut and medics, intending to cause chemical changes in the mind, often provoke gastro-intestinal issues, such as irritable bowel syndrome, as a side effect. Antidepressant medications (SSRIs), initially believed to be the cure for depression, change brain chemistry and contributed to chaos in the gut. As serotonin also plays a key role in moving food down the gut, altering the gut function will create side effects such as nausea, diarrhoea and constipation. The reason for this is that the gut-brain possesses the same neural receptors as the brain in our head. Anti-depressants treat both brains so it is clear that improving gut health will positively affect brain health. So, if people have both psychiatric and behavioural disturbances, one of the first places to look is the gut.

SEROTONIN AND THE GUT

Serotonin is a neurotransmitter, primarily found in the gastrointestinal tract (GI tract), blood platelets and the central nervous system. It is popularly thought to be a contributor to feelings of wellbeing and happiness. Approximately 90 per cent of the human body's total serotonin is located in the GI tract, where it is used to regulate intestinal movements.

It always comes as a surprise when I ask my students in Mind Body Cleanse masterclasses where they believe serotonin to be manufactured in the body. They always reply, 'In the brain, of course!' It always amazes everybody when I state that in fact 95 per cent of serotonin is produced in the gut's enteric nervous system. The gut is responsible for producing about 30 neurotransmitters along with this important 'happy chemical' and it shows why the gut is so central to feeling happy.

In coming years psychiatry will need to expand its scope to treat the second brain in addition to the one on the shoulders. And in some cases, it would be more effective if the gut had a session on the therapist's couch, rather than the brain. We should not always blame depression in the brain on our life circumstances.

The gut – brain axis

Stress is thought to be among the most important stimuli monitored through the gut – brain axis (see also page 19). When the brain senses a major issue, such as anger or fear, or that it is late for an appointment, it naturally wants to solve the problem. In order to solve the issue the brain needs energy, which it mainly borrows from the gut. Through the sympathetic nerve fibres the gut is instructed to obey the brain. The gut reduces blood supply and saves energy from temporarily digesting food because of this perceived emergency situation.

This system is not designed for over-use forever. However, if the brain thinks that it is in an emergency for the long term, the overworked gut will respond with negative stimulus, which may include diarrhoea, loss of appetite and fatigue. And if this situation is not checked over time, the health of the gut will eventually suffer. A reduced blood supply and a thinner layer of mucus will weaken the gut walls. The immune cells that live in the gut wall begin to secrete large amounts of signal substances that make the gut brain increasingly sensitive and eventually may influence behaviour and lead to illness down the line.

Making changes

Over the years I have been amazed at how simple lifestyle and eating habits have influenced behavioural, psychiatric and emotional issues with my one-on-one clients. Often clients have been so toxic that it has been a struggle to make real positive health changes, which require modifications in lifestyle and eating habits, and it is often the smaller incremental changes that make all the difference.

Marcus was a case like this:

I am 45 now, and have been morbidly overweight for most of my life.

After several months of yoga and plenty of water to flush out my system Chris finally let me go on to his 12-Day Plan. I was reluctant because I didn't think I'd make it 12 days without meat, cheese, pasta or fried food. I cheated on Day 1 and had some salmon. Day 2, I craved meat or fish, but resisted. Day 3, no cravings and in fact I started enjoying my outrageously delicious and varied salads, my sprouting beans and lentils, my hummus, olive oil, raw garlic, lime, coriander and a slew of spices and other herbs. I completed each stage of the Cleanse looking forward to the next day of my adventure with healthy eating. Days 7, 8 and 9 I felt amazing and had no symptoms to cause me concern, and then back to a gentle weaning off liquid for the last three days.

I have so far lost 55lb from my highest weight last year. I wake up without back pain and have a spring in my step. I do my yoga and I feel euphoric all day. I can't even look at the food I used to love without my stomach turning. And the quality of my life at home and at work has improved considerably.

My goal is to lose another 110lb in five years, though at this rate I'll do that long before my birthday in 2018.

Marcus is one of hundreds of clients I have seen undergo a remarkable transformation in wellness after rebalancing their gut and following the 12-Day Plan. An important realisation for Marcus is that you are far more in control of how you feel by how you eat and lifestyle factors than you realise.

Things that can go wrong in the gut

While the Mind Body Cleanse method and 12-Day Plan are suited to those who want to optimise their health and wellness, it is also good for people who want to recover from gut-related conditions. Over the years I have been amazed at the increase in cases of gut-related problems among clients.

Irritable-bowel syndrome

Irritable-bowel syndrome is often characterised by a bloating or gurgling sensation in the gut – unpleasant. There is also an increased susceptibility to constipation and diarrhoea-like symptoms. Sufferers of IBS who seek out yoga and meditation speak of anxiety and depression as often being linked to their symptoms. Sadly, the medical profession can still dismiss patients with IBS all too easily because tests often show no visible damage to the gut.

Other diseases affecting the bowel include conditions such as Crohn's disease or ulcerative colitis. Sufferers also show increased rates of depression and anxiety.

Sluggish bowels

A bloated tummy is often a warning sign of a sluggish intestine. You may be able to mitigate against the effects of sluggish bowels by:

- Eating slowly.
- Chewing your food thoroughly. Poorly chewed food will sit and ferment in your gut. Chew each mouthful at least 30 times and never eat when you are stressed, as Gandhi said: 'Chew your liquid and drink your solids.'
- Drinking plenty of water between meals. Dehydration will cause fluid retention and this will lead to bloating. Drink a minimum of 2.5 litres of fresh filtered water every day.
- Trying not to drink and eat simultaneously as this will dilute the gastric medium and make your digestive process less efficacious. Rather, drink water 30 minutes before or 30 minutes after eating.
- Eating too many acidic foods. Rather, eat more alkaline foods. Aim to make 80 per cent of what you eat alkaline.
- Eating early in the evening. Digestion is at its peak in the morning and thereafter slows down. Badly digested food will sit in your gut.

Avoid eating before bedtime and make breakfast your biggest meal of the day.

Food intolerances, allergies and sensitivities

At a professional level I have been surprised at the number of clients who count allergies and food intolerances and sensitivities as serious issues.

There are two different types of reactions to food. One is delayed and the other is immediate. And while some are immune-related, not all reactions are immune-related.

Food intolerances   A food intolerance is the result of a deficiency in a digestive enzyme that makes it difficult to break down a food nutrient, like the lactose in dairy products. It is not the same as a food allergy, and you may experience the following symptoms:

- Indigestion
- Gas
- Bloating
- Cramping
- Flatulence
- Loose stools.

Food allergies   cause an immediate response after contact with the substance. A food allergy may be characterised by the following symptoms:

- Anaphylaxis
- Shortness of breath or asthma
- Skin rash
- Itching of the skin
- Hives.

Food sensitivities   are characterised by a delayed response to a food substance. Often a common healthy food may be at the root of this problem. Symptoms may include:

- Migraines
- Mental fog and fatigue
- Delayed onset of symptoms – this makes it difficult to identify the food sources responsible

- Skin rashes
- Irritable bowel syndrome (IBS).

The best way to identify whether you are food-sensitive or intolerant is to keep a diary and keep track of your symptoms and eliminate specific foods as part of your 12-Day Plan.

Leaky–gut syndrome

A healthy gut works in a very similar way to cheesecloth. While it keeps the larger food particles, parasites, pathogenic gut bacteria and yeasts out, it allows all of the good nutrients through. Problems occur when these pathogens and larger food particles slip through the cheesecloth-like membrane and trigger an immune response. As the immune system hunts along the gut border for anything it does not recognise, it attacks these pathogens and larger food particles. In individuals with a predisposition to autoimmune diseases, the increased work for the immune system leads to a type of deregulation that eventually becomes an autoimmune disease. This causes inflammation and sensitivities.

Why do people develop a leaky gut? This could occur for one or more of the following reasons:
- Stress
- Dietary choices
- Infections
- Low stomach acid
- Toxic exposure to preservatives and pesticides
- Antibiotics.

Leaky gut is one of the most controversial and significant conditions when we are looking at gut imbalances. It is the description of the underlying pathology of numerous diseases that we treat yet have failed to find a cure for. Gut 'hypermeability' or 'leaky gut' is a process that has only begun to be accepted as a real syndrome in medicine comparatively recently. Often the symptoms are very similar to those of food-sensitivity reactions.

IBS and migraines can both be activated by immune reactions to food that a person may be consuming on a daily basis. If not treated, leaky gut can lead to serious inflammatory disorders and malnutrition.

Common symptoms may include:

- Fatigue
- Indigestion
- Constipation
- Weight gain.

The 12-Day Plan will certainly help many of the issues related to a leaky gut; however, you may require a longer bespoke approach to cure your unique imbalances from your health-care practitioner if symptoms persist.

Coeliac disease and gluten sensitivity

If you have coeliac disease, eating wheat can damage the villi in the gut wall and can cause serious infections. It can also damage the nervous system. For children it can be more serious and can cause diarrhoea and stunted growth. Symptoms may range from nausea to anaemia. The most effective treatment is a gluten-free diet.

Those with non-coeliac gluten sensitivity (NCGS) can eat wheat without serious risk to their small intestine, but should eat wheat in moderation. This is because you can become sensitive to gluten without developing autoimmune coeliac disease. Many people who do the 12-Day Plan, which is gluten-free, notice their sensitivity when they cut out gluten for 12 days and note a general improvement in their wellbeing. Digestive problems, flatulence, painful joints and headaches clear up, while energy levels and the ability to concentrate generally improves.

Gluten is a sticky protein that gives bread products their fluffiness and chewiness and it is omitted from the 12-Day Plan. It is a mixture of proteins found in wheat and related grains, including barley, rye and oats.

The incidence of NCGS, wheat allergy and gluten ataxia is increasing in most areas of the Western world. This is due mainly to the higher content of gluten in bread and bakery products, due to the reduction of dough fermentation time.

People with NCGS may develop gastrointestinal symptoms, which resemble those of irritable bowel syndrome or wheat allergy, and a wide variety of non-gastrointestinal symptoms, such as headache, chronic fatigue, fibromyalgia, atopic diseases, allergies, neurological diseases or even psychiatric disorders.

FEELING FOGGY?

A protein from gluten, gliadorphin, interacts with opiate receptors in the brain, mimicking opiate drugs such as heroin and morphine. These compounds affect the temporal lobe – an area of the brain that is associated with speech and hearing comprehension. That is why you can feel fogged up after a sandwich, for example.

In the same way that gluten metabolises into an opiate-like substance, so does the protein casein found in milk and other dairy products. Just like morphine, it makes you feel happier, calmer and sleepier.

Acid reflux and indigestion

Gastro-oesophageal reflux disease is a common condition where acid from the stomach leaks out of the stomach and up into the oesophagus (gullet). The oesophagus is a long tube of muscle that runs from the mouth to the stomach.

Common symptoms include:

- Heartburn – burning chest pain or discomfort that occurs after eating
- Acid reflux – you may have an unpleasant taste in the mouth caused by stomach acid coming back up into your mouth
- Pain when swallowing (odynophagia).

The answer to curing heartburn and acid indigestion is to restore your natural gastric balance and function. Eating large amounts of processed foods and sugars will exacerbate acid reflux as it will upset the bacterial balance in your stomach and intestine. So, before you turn to medication, you need to look at your lifestyle and diet. Instead, eat a lot of vegetables and other high-quality, ideally organic, whole foods. Eliminate caffeine, alcohol and nicotine products, which can trigger symptoms.

Acid reflux can also be a mechanical issue, as the pressure from too much food, incompletely digested and sitting in the stomach, especially if consumed too soon before bedtime, pushes stomach acid up the gullet. This leads to a burning sensation and inflammation.

Medications that suppress stomach acid may make your immediate symptoms better, but they should never be used long term to manage your indigestion or reflux because they may have serious long-term negative health effects.

Digestive enzyme deficiencies

Wellness depends on the breakdown and absorption of nutrients from the foods we eat, and enzymes are responsible for breaking down the foods into small absorbable units.

Digestive enzyme deficiency causes may include:
- Stress
- Toxicity
- Imbalanced stomach pH
- Infection and inflammation
- Free-radical damage.

You can see how serious this condition can become. If you cannot digest food properly, you may suffer from nutrient deficiencies and dysbiosis, and your potential to develop leaky-gut syndrome and food sensitivities is high.

If your symptoms get better with supplementation, with 'Gorgeous Greens' for example (see page 104), you can assume that you had a deficiency to begin with.

Symptoms of digestive enzyme deficiency:
- Fullness after a meal
- Gas and flatulence about one hour after eating
- Undigested food in stool
- Weight loss or weight gain
- Deficiency of fat-soluble vitamins.

CHAPTER 4

Food: what we put into our bodies

'Most people eat too much. A quarter of what they consume feeds them, the other three-quarters feeds the doctors.'

EGYPTIAN PAPYRUS

Understanding what our bodies need

If you want to understand how to create optimal wellness in your life (via my Mind Body Cleanse system), not only will you have to understand what is happening at a deeper level in your gut, as seen in the previous chapter, but you will also need to understand what is on the end of your knife and fork. The types of food that you eat can actually turn on or off good or bad genes. For example, if you consistently consume burgers and fries, you will turn on genes that promote inflammation. But if you eat rice and steamed broccoli, you will activate anti-cancer genes.

Proteins

Both animal and vegetable proteins are vital for the body and are responsible for growth and repair. The word protein comes from the Greek word *protos*, which means 'of prime importance'. Every part of the development of a foetus is dependent on it. Protein helps to regulate blood-sugar levels and leptin, which is produced in the fat cells and tells the hypothalamus in the brain when we are full. Proteins prevent cravings and their amino acids help to repair the villi in the intestines. They also help to create the receptors on the cells that enable the cells to communicate.

Because we are unable to manufacture the essential nine amino acids ourselves, we have to take them in our diet. Without these amino acids, malnutrition soon sets in because the body does not store proteins in the same way that it stores fats and carbohydrates.

Proteins take far longer than carbohydrates to digest, break down and absorb, which helps to regulate the rate at which insulin is released, preventing an abrupt rise in blood-sugar levels. This reduces the risk of diabetes.

Meat, fish and eggs

The easiest way to make sure you get all of your amino acids into your body is to eat meat or fish. However, you can get them from a vegetarian diet provided you think carefully about what you eat. If you choose to take animal proteins they should be grass-fed or organic wherever possible, so that you can avoid eating antibiotics and growth hormones too. The practice of feeding grain to animals makes their body composition change, with an alteration in the balance of fatty acids in their bodies. On the other hand, the levels of linoleic acid, a fat that reduces the risk of cancer, obesity, diabetes and some immune disorders, are much higher in grass-fed animals. And this is more in tune with the grass-fed meat of our ancestors, so it is more natural for us.

As regards fish, I recommend that you opt for 'sustainably farmed' because most fish these days is now farmed, to some extent.

Eggs are also an excellent source of protein – organic eggs are best.

Ditch the dairy

I recommend that you cut out all dairy produce while you are on the 12-Day Plan. The protein casein is mucus-forming and inflammatory and interferes with the integrity of the gut and the absorption of nutrients from the gut into the bloodstream.

When pasteurised, the two main proteins in milk, casein and whey, are devoid of the enzymes that can assimilate these proteins. For many people these proteins are hard to digest and can lead to food sensitivities.

Furthermore, the sugar lactose in milk can lead to an intolerance to milk that causes gas, bloating and diarrhoea. Lactose intolerance, which is different to a food sensitivity in that it is not immune-mediated (see also page 49), can be felt immediately after consuming milk and is painful.

MILK ALTERNATIVES

Here are some ideas for other, non-dairy, forms of milk:
> Rice milk, though some brands contain gluten so be careful which you choose.
> Soy milk. I'm not a fan of this because it can interfere with the absorption of essential minerals and has been linked to thyroid issues.
> Nut milks. The best ones are home made, but if you buy them ready-made make sure that they are unsweetened.

> Coconut milks are nutrient-packed, but avoid any brands that contain carrageenan, a red seaweed derivative.
> Hemp milk is a great source of omega 3, but watch out for added sugar.

If you are concerned about your calcium intake (present in dairy milk), there is more easily assimilated calcium in cabbage juice than there is in homogenised, pasteurised milk. The whole foods included in the 12-Day Plan will give your body the calcium it needs. By avoiding grains containing gluten, you will not be consuming phytates, which interfere with the absorption of calcium. You will take in more nutrients from eating less food.

Vegetable-based proteins
Vegetable proteins also contain an element of carbohydrate, unlike animal proteins.

Beans   Ideally, use dried beans and soak them overnight, or for at least 12 hours, in water containing a little added lemon juice, before boiling them twice. This is done in order to remove the phylates, which can irritate the gut and interfere with its ability to digest minerals. Chia, pumpkin, sunflower and sesame seeds should be treated in the same way, but they may need less time to hydrate.

Soy protein comes in many forms, from unfermented raw beans to fermented tempeh cakes. In an optimal diet, fermented soy products are better than unfermented products. Unfermented soy products contain phytates, which hinder the absorption of key nutrients, enzyme inhibitors and haemagglutin in, which causes red blood cells to lump together.

Carbohydrates

The term 'carbohydrate' includes all the grains, fruits and vegetables, as well as pulses, beans and peas. For many of us, carbohydrates provide the most abundant energy and fuel source for our bodies. However, not all carbohydrates are created equal.

Fruits and vegetables fall into sub-groups: the ones that can be broken down more readily into monosaccharides are the easiest to process. These are carbohydrates in their simplest form. Disaccharides or polysaccharides include potatoes and all refined sugars. Avoid the latter group while you are on the 12-Day Plan.

The body requires a continual intake of carbohydrates to feed the brain, which uses glucose. However, glucose not used by the brain gets stored in the form of glycogen. Once the glycogen levels in both the liver and the muscles are filled, excess carbohydrates are converted into fat and stored in the adipose tissue.

Vegetables   Eating a variety of vegetables is key to promoting good health because:

- Green and leafy vegetables are packed with vitamin C, and we must eat them daily
- Root vegetables provide slow-release energy and antioxidants
- You need calcium and magnesium for contracting and relaxing muscles
- Magnesium is important for the movement of the intestines or peristalsis
- Calcium is needed for a healthy nervous system, bones and teeth and blood-clotting.

Always choose seasonal vegetables and eat a wide array of vegetables when you are on the 12-Day Plan because of their fibre content and their antioxidant capacity to repair the gut.

'For a healthy gut you require a combination of soluble and insoluble fibre.'

THE IMPORTANCE OF FIBRE

You need to include enough fibre in your diet to enable regular movement and to facilitate peristalsis, to prevent the waste matter being reabsorbed through the intestinal wall.

For a healthy gut you require a combination of soluble and insoluble fibres. Soluble fibres help you to feel full by attracting water and creating a gel-like substance during digestion. This slows the rate at which the sugars that are broken down in the body enter the bloodstream, thus regulating insulin response. This, in turn, reduces the harmful effects of insulin in the body such as weight gain and the accumulation of fat around the middle. Soluble fibres also interfere with the absorption of cholesterol.

Good sources of soluble fibre can be found in:
- Psyllium
- Flaxseeds
- Oats
- Nuts
- Lentils
- Beans
- Pears
- Oranges
- Cucumbers
- Celery
- Carrots
- Apples.

As your healthy gut function is gradually restored during the 12-Day Plan, you should include foods that are full of insoluble fibre. These give bulk to the stools and prevent constipation. Because these fibres do not dissolve in water they pass through the intestinal tract intact, promoting the passage of waste matter. Good sources of insoluble fibre can be found in:
- Brown rice
- Whole grains
- Dark leafy greens
- Broccoli
- Cabbage
- Carrots
- Celery
- Cucumbers

- Fruits
- Green beans
- Nuts
- Seeds
- Courgettes.

PESTICIDES

Pesticides are a worldwide problem, being poisons that are sprayed onto foods to kill insects – and they are contributing to high levels of toxicity in the human gut. Farmers use low levels so as not to harm us, but even low levels increase the risk of toxic exposure and are best avoided. If possible, buy organic vegetables and fruits, or give them a good rinse before you eat them. It's even more important to wash foods that have thin skins, such as grapes and berries.

The main culprits are:
> Peaches
> Apples
> Peppers
> Celery
> Nectarines
> Strawberries
> Cherries
> Kale
> Lettuce
> Carrots
> Pears.

ANTIOXIDANTS

Antioxidants are nutrients that protect us from cellular damage and stress. They prevent ageing in our skin, brain and heart. They are found in brightly coloured foods, especially the vegetables that are used in the 12-Day Plan.
> Betacarotene is the vegetable form of vitamin A and is found in all berries, cherries, beetroot, red cabbage, aubergines and tomatoes
> Vitamin C is found in broccoli, chard, citrus fruits, bell peppers, kiwi and kale

> Vitamin E is found in avocado, sesame, chia, sunflower and pumpkin seeds and most nuts that are allowed in the 12-Day Plan
> Selenium is found in macadamia nuts, walnuts, Brazil nuts, sunflower and pumpkin seeds
> Zinc is found in walnuts, almonds, mushrooms and cocoa.

Fruits   The fruits that you can eat on the 12-Day Plan are all easy for the body to break down and cause the least fermentation in the gut.
- Ripe temperate fruits, including apples, pears, peaches and berries, are preferable to unripe ones because you can digest them more easily

- All fruits are rich in protective antioxidants, which help to repel toxins and pathogenic substances
- The vitamin A in fruits found in the form of betacarotene is great for your skin
- B vitamins are responsible for energy production and are responsible for all functions in the brain, adrenal gland and thyroid, which stimulates metabolism.

Insulin

Meals and snacks high in carbohydrates generate a rapid rise in blood sugar. In order to adjust to this rise, insulin is secreted by the pancreas into the bloodstream to lower the levels of glucose. The issue here is that insulin is primarily a storage hormone, which evolved to store carbohydrate to prepare for periods of famine. As a result, fat accumulates where the insulin has been stimulated by excess carbohydrate. Therefore when we eat too much carbohydrate we send a signal to the body to store fat. This is a vicious circle because insulin also prevents the body from releasing stored fat.

Worse still, insulin also causes feelings of hunger. As blood sugar increases following a carbohydrate meal, insulin rises, with the result of lowered blood sugar. This will result in hunger after just an hour or so. This vicious circle leads to unhealthy snacking and weight gain and also to energy crashes and irritability.

Insulin responses vary from person to person, but to stop this cycle of spikes and crashes, you have to moderate your intake of grains and refined sugars. Refined carbohydrates do not have the natural fibre that helps to minimise the carbohydrate/insulin response.

Another problem with insulin is that over time our bodies can develop insulin-resistance, often known as 'metabolic syndrome', which can develop into diabetes. Here are some of the symptoms associated with metabolic syndrome:
- Fatigue
- Brain 'fog' and poor memory
- Low blood sugar
- Bloating

- Sleepiness
- Weight gain
- Increased triglycerides
- Increased blood pressure
- Depression.

There are many sources of sugar that are hidden in our normal diets, and the 12-Day Plan excludes them.

During the 12-Day Plan you will need to cut out refined grains, which make up many of the cereals, biscuits and cakes that we tend to include in our Western diets. These foods are most damaging to the gut lining, along with coffee and alcohol.

Refined sugars

Refined sugars are empty calories and contain no nutritional value. Furthermore, sugar is also toxic to the body and its over-consumption wreaks havoc with our immune and endocrine systems. Studies show that sugar is just as habit-forming as any narcotic. When you consume a refined carbohydrate your body 'borrows' vital nutrients such as calcium, sodium, potassium and magnesium from healthy cells in order to metabolise this incomplete food. In a worst-case scenario bones can become osteoporotic due to the calcium withdrawal.

Many people in the West eat large amounts of sugar and grains, which generate large quantities of insulin circulating in the blood. Initially, sugar satisfies the craving centres in the brain, increases your blood pressure and heart rate, and can give you the feeling of an energy surge. But soon your insulin levels start to rise to stabilise and control the blood-sugar level, and as a result you can start to feel irritable and angry. You can also feel drowsy, perhaps with headaches too. If you are particularly toxic you may feel the effect in your muscles and joints. An hour to two hours after your sugar hit, your sugar levels drop low enough that your body kicks into high gear. Cortisol is secreted to stabilise your blood sugar and maintain homeostasis. The cortisol triggers your adrenals and you may feel panicky and anxious. Soon your brain is demanding another sugar hit. This vicious cycle is like a roller coaster. The higher you go up, the harder you crash afterwards.

When you stop eating theses foods, your body can take several days to lower your insulin levels. In the meantime, the high insulin levels prompt symptoms such as headaches, dizziness and confusion. In the first few days of the 12-Day Plan, you can eat protein and fibre to help counteract this, and drink plenty of water. Don't give up hope, you can easily detox from sugar-laden foods, and the 12-Day Plan is designed to help you to do just that.

Why sugar is bad for you

Sugar has a negative impact on the body because it:

- Causes insulin resistance, which can lead to heart and vascular disease, diabetes
- Causes inflammation, a major precursor to disease, and a fatty liver linked to obesity, especially in children
- Is highly addictive
- Raises your cholesterol
- Is unsustainable energy and devoid of essential minerals, nutrients and fatty acids
- Is linked to a decrease in the intake of essential micronutrients.

THE ADDICTIVE NATURE OF PROCESSED GOODS

Did you know that your food choices are not all under your control? The food industry has preyed on our brain chemistry by researching and designing the combination of salt, sweet and fat that make foods so addictive that it is incredibly difficult to stop eating (or drinking) after just one bite or sip. Deceptive labelling has exacerbated the problem.

Processed foods also cause damage to our internal organs and make our brains crave more. This is a vicious cycle. One of the most common cravings is sugar and you may eat too much sugar without realising it because it is hidden in all sorts of so-called 'healthy' foods or food-like products. For example, cereals may be labelled and advertised as being 'healthy', even though they are actually laden with refined sugars.

Sugar may be hidden in the following processed foods:

> Low-fat and 'diet' foods often contain extra sugar to help improve their taste and palatability and to add bulk and texture in place of fat
> Savoury, seemingly 'healthy' foods, such as ready-made soups and sauces, may contain added sugar
> A can of soft drink, on average, contains the equivalent of seven teaspoonfuls of sugar.

You can check the level of sugar in your food in the following ways:

Look at the 'carbs as sugars' section on the nutrition panel of the product label. This lists both natural and added sugars. Less than 5g per 100g is low; more than 22.5g per 100g is high. (continued)

The higher up the ingredients list anything ending in 'ose', such as glucose, sucrose, fructose, lactose, maltose, is, the more sugar the product contains.

While xylitol, sorbitol and mannitol can be used as substitutes for sugar, they can still send confusing messages to the brain and maintain a degree of dependency on sugary sweetness. Beware – many health and wellness brands use these ingredients to make their 'healthy' products taste better! Therefore it is best to cut out refined sugars and sugar substitutes entirely.

The only way to break the sugar cycle is to stop eating these foods and you can easily do this by doing the 12-Day Plan.

Fats

Fat is the most efficient and valuable food particle. Its atoms are combined in such a way that they concentrate twice as much energy per gram as carbohydrates or protein. Fats provide the best source of energy for the body and are not simply a curse to the waistline, as we once thought – they are healthy when they come from whole, natural, unprocessed foods.

While it is important to understand that not all fats are created equal, it is also vital to understand fat's vital functions. They create sex hormones such as oestrogen and testosterone, adrenal hormones such as cortisol and steroid hormones, and the neurological system depends on the intake of good fats.

The benefits of including the right fats include improved mood, focus and ability to concentrate, good skin, lustrous, soft hair, as well as improving the immune function through fat-soluble nutrients such as vitamin A, D, E and K.

- Fats are essential to brain function and the brain is composed 60 per cent of fats
- 60 per cent of our heart's energy comes from fat
- Fats in a meal slow down the digestive process
- Fats protect the myelin sheath that insulates nerve fibres, just like the plastic covering on an electric cable
- Lungs need a high concentration of fats to enable the lungs to expand and function effectively, allowing the body to breathe.

Fat is unique. Unlike other nutrients it cannot be absorbed directly into the blood from the gut because it is insoluble in water. Fat has a different route of assimilation into the body: it is absorbed via the lymphatic system. Fat converges at the thoracic duct, skirts the belly and heads straight for the heart, without inspection by the liver, unlike other food particles. Detoxification of bad fat only takes place after it has been pumped through the system, and this is precisely why some types of fat can have an extremely harmful negative effect at the level of the body.

Conversely, 'good' fat can work wonders. Cold-pressed virgin olive oil, for example, can protect against arteriosclerosis, cellular stress, Alzheimer's and eye disease. Good fat also has a positive effect on inflammatory diseases such as rheumatoid arthritis.

There are three main types of fat:
- Saturated fat is found in butter and animal fat, ghee, palm oil and coconut oil
- Monosaturated fat is found in avocado oil, olive oil and almonds
- Polyunsaturated fat is found in fish oil, flaxseed oil, sesame oil, walnut oil and corn.

Saturated fats
Saturated fats used to be considered unhealthy as it was thought that they could increase the level of bad, low-density lipoprotein (LDL) cholesterol in the blood and arteries, which may contribute to heart disease and stroke. However, we now know that it is the combination of fats and sugars that creates arterial plaque. Saturated fat is rich in linoleic acid (CLA), which helps to break down fat stored in the body.

Saturated fats:
- Contribute to 50 per cent of the phospholipid component of cell membranes that gives our cells integrity
- They play a vital role with our bones and their mineral density
- They enhance the immune system and protect us against harmful microorganisms in the digestive tract
- They protect the liver from alcohol and other toxins.

Monosaturated fats

These fats are semi-solid when chilled. They contribute to heart health as well as reducing plaque by stimulating the release of bile. These fats are rich in flavour.

Sources of monosaturated fat:

- Olive oil
- Avocado
- Macadamia nut oils (these oils should be used in a cold-pressed state for salad dressings only).

Polyunsaturated fats

Polyunsaturated fats are more vulnerable to oxidation or hydrogenation, and if not used properly have many negative health implications. This is why it is important to store your oils in a cool place, out of the sun, with the lid completely closed.

High heat and chemicals used by manufacturers to process oils are the chief sources of damaged fats. One particularly damaging process is partial hydrogenation, which gives oils a longer shelf life. This process creates trans fats and other altered molecules. Trans fatty acids increase risk of coronary heart disease by raising levels of 'bad' LDL cholesterol and lowering levels of good cholesterol. Trans fatty acids have also been linked to degenerative diseases, inflammation, acceleratory ageing, Alzheimer's, cancer, diabetes, obesity and infertility.

ESSENTIAL FATS

The two main groups of essential fats – omega 3 and omega 6 – are essential because the body cannot manufacture them itself, so we have to acquire them from the food we eat. Both groups complement each other in their benefits, yet both are required to balance each other out. The ratio of omega 3 to omega 6 is important for the synthesis of prostaglandins. Prostaglandins from omega 6 promote cell proliferation, inflammation and blood clotting, whereas prostaglandins from omega 3 do the opposite. This is why the balance between the two is so crucial: we want our blood to have clotting qualities, but we also want it to flow freely.

> These fats are essential for brain, heart and cardiovascular health
> Omega 3s are found in fish oil, flaxseed oil, hemp seeds, herring, sardines, walnuts, algae and egg yolk

(continued)

> Omega 6s, typically found in the American diet, is found in corn oil, grapeseed oil, sesame oil, soybean oil and meat.

People who thrive on a low-fat diet and lack of omega 3s are prone to arthritis and inflammatory conditions such as eczema and psoriasis. They can also suffer from poor memory, depression, hair loss, liver and kidney degeneration, and behavioural disturbances.

These fats can be found in nuts and seeds – this source of omega 3 is less easy for your body to absorb and use than animal derived fats. However, for the purpose of the 12-Day Plan, it is best to go vegan, therefore eating meat during the Plan is not advised. Omega 3 also helps create serotonin, which is synthesised in the gut.

CHOLESTEROL

Cholesterol has gained a reputation as something to be avoided, but this view is no longer held. High-density lipoprotein (HDL), also known as 'good' cholesterol, is one of the main groups of lipoproteins that transport fats and cholesterol in the blood. A high level of HDL seems to protect against heart disease.

Low-density lipoprotein or 'bad cholesterol' transports cholesterol and fats back to the liver to be processed, like HDL. LDL transports cholesterol from the liver out to the tissues. Owing to this, a high level of LDL is a marker for cardiovascular disease.

CHAPTER 5
Yoga and intelligent movement

The history and legacy of yoga

Yoga has been described as the cessation of the fluctuations of the mind or the state of inner felt union achieved when the mind is still. As such, yoga and meditation form the backbone of the Mind Body Cleanse system in this book. When I started my yoga journey in India, I practised a form of yoga called 'kriya' yoga. The term 'kriya' in yoga has become synonymous with the system of inner-cleansing techniques discussed in this chapter. It is the practical branch of yoga that can lead to a change for the better in all aspects of our lives. It is the 'yoga of action', the means by which we achieve yoga as a state of being.

'Kriya is the "yoga of action", the means by which we achieve yoga as a state of being.'

The yoga sutra defines kriya yoga as being made up of three components: tapas, svadhyaya and isvarapranidhana.

Tapas
'Tapas', meaning 'to burn or create heat', is something we do in order to keep us physically and mentally healthy. It is a process of inner cleansing: we remove what we do not need and whatever is burned out is purified in the same way that the more you fire gold, the purer it becomes. However, this is not the same as mortification or austerity.

AN EXAMPLE OF TAPAS – OR PERHAPS NOT?

I remember when I was in the Himilaya at Gangotri, near the source of the Ganga, where many holy men live, I came across a group of Sadhus who practised austerity in the name of yoga. One man had his arm raised, apparently a widely known phenomenon, and it had withered horribly, his fingers were blackened, his fingernails lengthened. Someone told me that this arm had been raised like this for 36 years.

KRIYA YOGA

Kriya yoga is the practical branch of yoga that can lead to a change for the better in all aspects of our lives. It is the yoga of action and is the means by which we achieve yoga as a state of being.

Svadhyaya is the process of gradually finding out where we are, who we are, what we are and so forth. We can take this step by observing the breath and body. We do this again and again, hoping that we will, with time, develop a deeper understanding of ourselves and our current state. In this way we can identify what our next steps will be. This close connection holds true for every kind of yoga practice.

However, Svadhyaya is not just 'study', per se, but study of the true self, rather than mere analysis of the mind. Anything that will elevates the mind and reminds you of your true self should be studied: the Bible, the Koran or the Bhagavad Gita.

Studying means studying with your heart, not just passing over the pages.

If you want to understand me fully, you must become me.

The self cannot just be known by theory alone. By merely thinking, no one has ever understood anything that is beyond the mind. Only when you transcend the mind can you understand it. This is where yoga differs from most other psychological approaches, in which you usually have to understand everything with the mind – beyond it you cannot understand anything.

The literal meaning of isvarapranidhana is 'to yield humbly to God'. The meaning in the context of kriya yoga relates to a special kind of attention to action: we place value on the quality of our action, not on the resultant fruits of our action. We therefore pay attention to the spirit with which we act and look less to the results our actions may bring us – indeed, the more distanced we are from the fruits of our labour, the better we are able to do this. We then bypass the tendency to set ourselves up for failure. We should remain flexible, and not just in our yoga asanas.

Cross-fertilisation

One of the most exciting developments in the last 50 years is the cross-fertilisation of Western science with ideas from ancient Eastern wisdom systems such as yoga. With increasing precision, scientists are able to look at the brain and body and detect the sometimes-subtle changes that practitioners of yoga and meditation undergo. In former times, few yoga studies were carried out in the West, and most scientists dismissed Indian yoga research due to methodological problems, such as a lack of study control groups. Now methodology is much improved and it could be argued that many Indian studies of yoga are superior to most of those done in the West. In fact, more people practise Hatha yoga in California then they do in India.

As yoga becomes more and more mainstream in the West, and as complementary health systems continue to grow, studies of yoga are getting not only better but also more numerous in both India, Europe and the United States. In just the last few years, research has documented the efficacy of yoga for such conditions as back pain, multiple sclerosis, insomnia, cancer, heart disease, gut-related problems and even tuberculosis. Studies are also increasingly documenting how yoga works. Among its many beneficial effects, yoga has been shown to increase strength, flexibility and balance; enhance immune function; lower blood sugar and cholesterol levels; and improve psychological wellbeing. One of yoga's most prominent effects, of course, is stress reduction (see also page 19).

The Mind Body Cleanse methods discussed in Part 2 (in the 12-Day Plan) require us to be aware of our bodies. Yoga asanas, pranayama and meditation begin to break down the distance from our inner selves and bring us into close contact with our sensations and feelings. Knowing how our bodies really feel, we can notice when we are stressed and can make decisions about our activities and our attitudes that can influence our actions and relationships.

Stress and the autonomic nervous system

Although yoga is so much more than a method of stress-reduction – and stress certainly adversely affects a wide range of health conditions – yoga is arguably one of the most comprehensive approaches to fighting stress and alleviating its symptoms. Stress isn't just a factor in conditions commonly labelled 'stress-related', such as migraines, ulcers and irritable bowel syndrome, but it appears to contribute to such major killers as heart attacks, diabetes and osteoporosis. Even for diseases such as cancer, yoga can improve not only the quality of life after diagnosis, but it appears to diminish the side effects of surgery, radiation, chemotherapy and other treatments, and may increase the odds of survival.

Fight and flight/rest and relaxation

For the purposes of this book, we are most interested in the effects of stress at the level of the gut and our elimination and detoxification systems. And to appreciate the role of stress in this, it's important to understand the function of the autonomic nervous system (ANS), which controls the function of the heart, liver, intestines and other internal organs. The ANS has two branches that work in conjunction with each other: the sympathetic nervous system (SNS) or 'flight and fight', and the parasympathetic nervous system (PNS) or 'rest and relaxation' response.

Sympathetic and parasympathetic are anatomically separate but most organs are supplied by neurones from both (e.g. heart, lung, gut). Some organs are just affected by sympathetic (e.g. the adrenal gland to release adrenaline, liver to release glucose). Some organs are only stimulated by the parasympathetic system (e.g. kidney).

The SNS, in conjunction with such stress hormones as adrenaline and cortisol, help you deal with a crisis situation. The PNS, by contrast, tends to slow the heart, lower blood pressure, and can be thought of as 'rest and digest'.

During periods of relaxation, when the parasympathetic branch of the autonomic nervous system takes over the digestive, elimination and sexual systems are activated. For men, the production of testosterone occurs while in a state of relaxation. There are some serious implications for fertility here.

Mind Body Cleanse techniques, including yogic asanas, in conjunction with slow breathing, meditation, guided imagery and cleansing lead to an increase in the activation of the PNS, mental relaxation and good gut function.

Intelligent movement

The Mind Body Cleanse system incorporates 'intelligent movement', which is the system of yoga and coordinated breath work outlined in the 12-Day Plan.

'We have lost our connection with the rhythm of life and with our own internal rhythms and the rhythm of our own body mind.'

As I have developed my yoga and life practice, I have become convinced that as we humans have become increasingly more 'civilised', we have forgotten how to listen to our instinctual self. The net effect is that we have become distanced from our physical bodies. We have lost our connection with the rhythm of life and with our own internal rhythms and the rhythm of our own body mind.

We now find ourselves eating compulsively, serving our desires and emotions, rather than what is wholesome and nourishing. When we are 'present' in our lives, when we listen to our intuition, we know what to eat and how to eat it; we are no longer hostages to a world of fast food and half-truths about what's good for us – we know what the body needs and we eat to satisfy it rather than our emotions and compulsions.

Research has shown that movement is good for your heart, for building lean muscle, for improving metabolism, and for balancing moods and lowering stress hormones. New science is showing us that movement also benefits the gut and so too the microbiome – that diverse ecosystem living inside comprising trillions of symbiotic bacteria (see page 35). Intelligent movement can help you to quieten your mind, so that you can feel and then release the tension stored in your gut.

For many, 'exercise' means going to the gym for 45 minutes three times a week, with perhaps a mix of treadmill and high-resistance weight training. Unfortunately, this approach is unenlightened in the long term as it can over-stress joints, split muscle fibres and result in the development of scar tissue. What is needed is a varied approach to movement. This book shows you how the Mind Body Cleanse practice sequence, as part of my 12-Day Plan, is an intelligent form of movement consisting of yoga and coordinated breath work. It can help you to reconnect with your body and mind, and will help you to experience a different way of moving and relating to your internal organs that will help you tune in to what is good for your mind and body.

'Intelligent movement', consisting of yoga and coordinated breath work, is great therapy on all levels. First, it can be a wonderful way of reducing stress, especially when practised with good breathing techniques. Second, you can become more flexible and stronger, though it's important to be aware that the practice is not meant to be competitive in any sense, either with others or with yourself, which is sometimes hard for Westerners to take on board. Internally, the Mind Body Cleanse intelligent-movement sequence stimulates detoxification and metabolism, while mentally it establishes awareness and clarity plus a confident and calm sense of self. Moreover, the technique is a dialogue with your body. And through this

'When we are "present" in our lives, when we listen to our intuition, we know what to eat and how to eat it.'

'Intelligent movement can help you to quieten your mind, so that you can feel and then release the tension stored in your gut.'

dialogue you can develop a deeper awareness of it so that you know when you can push a little further and when you can rest.

Start wherever you are

My teacher in India used to tell me that you can start your practice wherever you are now. This means that you accept wherever you are now. And this includes sickness or injury. When you move with this understanding, you switch on your parasympathetic branch of the autonomic nervous system (PNS); your rest and relaxation response. When the PNS is activated through the 12-Day Plan, your stomach, liver, pancreas and gall bladder secrete acidic and alkaline juices and hormones to promote healthy digestion. Research has shown that the natural balance of healthy bacteria in the gut can be affected positively by this.

So when you eat on the run, or 'inhale' your food at your desk, you are eating with your flight-or-fight response switched on, or the sympathetic branch of the autonomic nervous system. Your blood flow is shunted away from the digestive system, so your gut slows down and comes to a halt. This is useful in an emergency, when you need to increase blood circulation and oxygen to be directed into your arms, legs and brain for a speedy response. However, when the flight-or-fight response is prolonged, your abdominal muscles contract and peristalsis comes to a halt, resulting in constipation, abdominal pain and gut disorder.

'The 12-Day Plan helps to connect your mind to your body and your gut.'

Using the breathing and meditation techniques listed in the 12-Day Plan you can trigger the PNS to give your body a natural state of balance. Through the Plan sequence you can change your focus towards health and connection and instantly begin the process of healing and disease resolution. This is the mind – body – gut relationship that you want to create. The 12-Day Plan helps to connect your mind to your body and your gut.

When these three elements (mind, body and gut) are fully connected, you awaken a deeper connection to your authentic self; to the inner knowing of things that are not learned but are an innate part of you, encoded in your DNA: your real human nature. In this connected state you can begin to care for yourself and stop abusing your own body.

Sadly, in the modern world the trinity of the mind – body – gut is poorly understood and supported. To begin with, our eating habits have deteriorated. We have lost our Sundays, in which we traditionally had a day of rest, gathering for a family meal, and participating in other activities that allowed us to relate to each other and listen deeply to one another. And with the advent of the Internet and widespread use of social media, we have begun to ignore the body further while the mind is ceaselessly connected to the white noise of technology. We have begun to lose our human touch. It is clear that our lives need to be returned to balance; we need to slow down, take leisure seriously, learn how to switch off, relate to each other better, get better work/life balance, listen to the body, get enough sleep, learn how to cook and make time for it, eat wholesome food, take time for exercise, vacation and regular downtimes.

The yoga poses described in Part 2 are designed to let us remember the body and listen to its intelligence. However, they are not meant be a substitute for yoga classes, if you attend them. If you are new to yoga, I recommend attending introductory classes or private sessions prior to starting the 12-Day Plan. The poses are a guide to those who already have a semi-regular practice but who want to make it more regular. A home practice can help you delve a little deeper into your yoga and create consistency. As we progress through the 12 days of the Plan, I will continue to add poses to your yoga practice – but feel free to add other poses as you like. Ideally, this home practice is meant to be done on the days when you can't make it to a full yoga class.

And remember, when you are listening sensitively to your body, you will notice that its responses are continuous, which means that you will be able to engage at a different level with the world, and you will become more sensitive to the goings-on around you.

Twists to help gut health

Twisting poses, which you will be using as part of the 12-Day Plan, when combined with the breath, teach the importance of a healthy spine and inner body. The action of a twist squeezes and flushes the pelvic and abdominal organs with fresh blood – a 'squeeze-and-soak' action. As the organs compress, blood filled with metabolic byproducts and toxins is pushed out. When we release the twist, fresh blood flows in, carrying oxygen and the essential building blocks for tissue healing.

Twists are quite remarkable because they not only massage, tone and rejuvenate your abdominal organs and promote digestion and peristalsis, but also improve the suppleness of the diaphragm and relieve spine, hip and groin disorders. The spine also becomes more supple, allowing for the correct spacing and alignment in between the spinal vertebrae. This in turn improves the flow of blood to the spinal nerves and increases energy levels. (See pages 130–3, 146–51 and 182 for twists.)

Twists for living younger longer

Spinal rotation is important for posture and structural alignment. However, many people lose full spinal rotation because of living a sedentary lifestyle, because they do not move around enough and spend a lot of time sitting at a desk. Some movement losses occur if joints fuse due to trauma, surgery or arthritis, but most loss comes from the shortening of soft tissues. If you don't work the muscles, tendons, ligaments and connective tissues fully at least a few times a week, they will gradually shorten and limit the joints' mobility. In the case of twisting, the limitation is usually in soft tissues around the upper or lower spine.

If you regularly practise twists, there are clear benefits for your joints and soft tissue – you maintain the normal length and resilience of the soft tissues and help to maintain the health of the discs and of the facet joints. This will help to maintain good posture and structural alignment into your old age without gravity making a negative effect.

As you twist, the layers of muscle and bone revolve deeply; your attention is drawn into the stable, unmoving centre of the pose. This ability to stay centred, as the hubbub of the world swirls around you like around the eye of the storm, will help you live your life more calmly and serenely.

Anatomy of twists   There are a few anatomical points to keep in mind with twists. Most important is to elongate your spine with the inhalation; a slumped-over posture significantly limits spinal rotation. So before you start the twist, take a moment to ground your sitting bones and draw your spine straight up towards the crown of your head. Make sure that your spine is perpendicular to the floor, rather than listing to the side, front or back.

Each section of the spine has a different rotational mobility. The cervical (neck) vertebrae, for example, are the most mobile in twisting. Because the 12 thoracic (mid-back) vertebrae have ribs attached, they can't twist as freely as the neck vertebrae. And because of the orientation of the lumbar (lower spine) facet joints, the rotation of these five vertebrae is the most limited. Each time you move into a twisting posture, be conscious that you don't over-twist in the more mobile areas.

To ensure that you don't over-twist at your neck, begin your seated twist by bringing your awareness into your tummy, and begin the twist from there – as if you were using your abdominal obliques to twist your body around. Let the twist gradually unfold up your spine, as though you were walking up a spiral staircase, so that each vertebra participates in the twist. If you twist quickly and without awareness, your neck will likely do most of the twisting and whole sections of your spine can remain stuck. Rather, keep your chin in line with your mid-chest. It's easy to turn your head around your shoulders, but it's certainly a lot more challenging and beneficial to twist your upper body around your lower body.

Muscle activity   Many muscle groups are involved in twists, contracting and shortening or stretching and lengthening. There are several groups of back muscles of varying length: the rotators, semispinalis and multifidus all contribute to spinal rotation. Some of the muscles that actively rotate the torso are quite small, like the intercostals, the layers of muscle between each two ribs. And several sets of muscles contribute to your ability to turn your head; the easiest to see is the sternocleidomastoid. The two SCMs sit on the front of your neck, forming a 'V' starting at the top of the breastbone and running to the base of the skull just behind each ear. Look in a mirror: if you turn your head to the right, you'll see your left SCM contract, and vice versa.

Probably the most important muscle group in active twisting are the abdominal obliques. The obliques form two layers of muscle on either side of the better-known rectus abdominus, the 'six-pack' muscle that runs vertically up the centre of the abdomen from the pubic bone to the ribcage. The two internal obliques, left and right, originate primarily from the pelvis and travel diagonally up across the abdomen, while the two external obliques originate primarily from the lower ribcage and travel diagonally down across the abdomen. All of the obliques have strong attachments to the substantial fascia of the lower back and to the gut.

Taken together, the four obliques form a diagonal cross that girdles the abdomen and they have important functions in supporting the lower back, pelvis and internal organs. The diagonal lines of the muscles also give them strong leverage in rotating the torso. When you turn to the right in Bharadvaja's Twist (see page 148), for example, the left external oblique will team with the right internal oblique to rotate your torso. At the same time, the opposite pair of obliques will have to lengthen. (And so your twisting range of motion can be reduced by the inability of one pair – one external oblique and the other opposite internal oblique – to lengthen, while weakness in the opposite pair could limit your ability to actively draw yourself into the twist).

Benefits to your consciousness of twists

Like any yoga posture, you should practise twists with mindfulness and care. Remember the following principles as you move through them.

- **Let the breath be your guide.** Because twists tend to compress the diaphragm, they leave you with little breathing room. But there are ways to let your breath support and guide you through your twisting explorations. Here's one approach: as you inhale, lengthen the spine; as you exhale, revolve gently into your twisting posture. Pause and lengthen again on the next inhalation, then rotate further as you exhale. Continue breathing and moving in this wave-like fashion until you feel you've nestled into the depths of the pose. Breathe as steadily and rhythmically as possible for several breaths, then slowly come out of the pose.
- **Practise evenly on both sides.** Because twists are asymmetrical postures, it's a good idea to spend equal time revolving in each direction to promote balance. That said, if you know that one side of your body is tighter than the other, you might try doing a twist for longer on that side.
- **Enjoy the after-effects.** Don't miss out on the opportunity to enjoy the sensations of clarity, vitality and ease once you've emerged from your favourite twist.

Finally, you may have heard that a *'twist a day keeps old age at bay ...'* well, there is good reason to say this! To maintain or restore the normal spinal rotation, I recommend that you practise a simple spinal twice a day.

Inversions for fighting gravity

The ancient yogis called gravity 'the silent enemy'. Gravity has a profound effect on the physiological processes of the human body; it slowly but surely weighs us down and saps our strength. We stand, sit or walk with the head above the heart, and the legs and pelvis beneath. But as the years rack up, so do the damages. Subcutaneous fat sags, varicose veins appear and, finally, the heart can become overworked.

There are four major systems in the body that the practice of inversions is said to positively influence: cardiovascular, lymphatic, nervous and endocrine systems. In particular, the lymphatic system is responsible for waste removal, fluid balance and immune system response. Lymph vessels arise among the capillary beds of the circulatory system, but comprise a separate system that transports stray proteins, waste materials and extra fluids, filtering the fluid back through the lymph nodes and dumping what remains into the circulatory system at the subclavian veins, under the collarbones.

Lymph, like the blood returning to your heart via the veins, is dependent upon muscular movement and gravity to facilitate its return. Because the lymphatic system is a closed pressure system and has one-way valves that keep lymph moving towards the heart, when you turn upside down the entire lymphatic system is stimulated, thus strengthening your immune system, relaxing the gut and stimulating the elimination system too.

To receive these palpable benefits, and to prevent injury, it's essential to learn the correct setup and alignment for each pose – so learn the poses from a qualified teacher first before you practise them at home.

When I first started practising yoga in India, my teacher told me that a yoga practice without inversions is like 'marriage without wife'. And I have since been drawn to inversions for two simple reasons – they make my body feel good and they're fun. They bring out my inner sense of adventure and playfulness.

CONTRAINDICATIONS

If you have a spinal disc injury, consult your health-care provider before practising twists of any kind.

Practise one of the seated twists every day during the 12-Day Plan, and for full spinal movement into old age I recommend a daily twist for the rest of your life!

Psychologically, inversions allow us to see things from an alternative perspective and they require stability and awareness. They make you feel stable as well. One feeds into the other. Emotionally, they guide the energy of the pelvis, the kernel of creation and personal power, towards the heart centre, enabling self-exploration and inner growth. Physically, they stimulate the immune and endocrine systems, thereby invigorating and nourishing the brain and the internal organs. When done correctly, inversions also release tension in the neck and spine.

Until very recently, there was little interest in the West in objectively documenting the effects of inversions on health, but now the benefits of inversions are built on expert opinion, case studies and educated reasoning. We can cite biomechanical principles, measure indices such as heart rate or blood pressure, and witness the effects of inversions on people who practise regularly.

'I have been practising a 10-minute head balance every day for the last 12 years. Its therapeutic application has helped me enormously with maintaining a healthy blood pressure and weight. I also feel confident and relaxed throughout the day as a result. The area around my neck and shoulders has definitely strengthened, as well as my core strength. I have a very stressful job and I swear by the benefits of this one yogic pose.'

All the evidence points to one principal, galvanising effect that inversions have on the practitioner – they change your relationship to gravity.

In a 1992 *Yoga International* article on headstands and the circulatory system, Coulter, Master of Anatomy and Physiology, wrote: 'If you can remain in an inverted posture for just 3 to 5 minutes, the blood will not only drain quickly to the heart, but tissue fluids will flow more efficiently into the veins and lymph channels of the lower extremities and of the abdominal and pelvic organs, facilitating a healthier exchange of nutrients and wastes between cells and capillaries.'

Finally, inverting gives your heart a break. The heart works to ensure that freshly oxygenated blood makes its way up to your brain and its sensory organs. When you are inverting, the pressure differential across your body is reversed and blood floods the carotid arteries in the neck. It is believed that baroreceptors, mechanisms that calibrate blood flow to the brain, sense the increase in blood, and slow the flow, thus reducing blood pressure and heart rate. It has not, however, been clinically established whether the practice of inversion could lower blood pressure in the long term and, in fact, high blood pressure is typically considered to be a contraindication for inversions. But this depends on the individual, and each person is different.

To receive these palpable benefits and to prevent injury, especially to the neck, it's essential to be taught, and therefore to learn, the correct setup and alignment for each inverted pose. Also, I recommend that women don't do inversions during menstruation; reversing blood flow goes against the body's natural urge to release stale blood and the endometrial lining, and it may lead to a backflow of menstrual fluid known as 'retrograde menstruation'. Other contraindications include neck injuries, epilepsy, high blood pressure, heart conditions and eye problems. So be mindful about your body as you approach these poses.

Forward bends

Forward bends are important in the Mind Body Cleanse because, during forward bends, your abdominal organs are compressed and this has a unique effect on your nervous system as these organs relax, your frontal brain is cooled and the flow of blood to your entire brain is regulated. Your sympathetic nervous system is rested, bringing down your pulse rate and blood pressure. The adrenal glands are also soothed and they function more efficiently. Since your body is in a horizontal position in forward bends, your heart is relieved of the strain of pumping blood against gravity, and blood circulates through all parts of the body easily. Forward bends also strengthen the para-spinal muscles, inter-vertebral joints and ligaments.

Forward bends can be wonderfully relaxing and make you feel pleasantly introspective; however, they can also strain or injure your lower back, especially if the backs of your legs are tight, so you need to be careful.

Learning to practise forward bends correctly means that you must pay close attention to the mechanics of your body. The crucial muscles to understand are the hamstrings, particularly in their interactions with your pelvis. When the hamstrings are pushed to the limit of their flexibility, they rebel and avoid further stretching by either bending the knee or extending the hip. The tighter your hamstrings are, the more likely it is that this will happen. And that can be bad news for your back. It is important, therefore, that you keep your back straight during forward bends.

If you have been attending yoga classes already, you may have heard your teacher tell you to contract your quadriceps (the muscles on the front of your thighs) in forward bends. If your hamstrings are tight, this is an excellent way to help them loosen up. The quads will stabilise your knees and hold them straight in forward bends while the hams try to cheat and bend the knees. Not only that, but by contracting your quads, you'll be taking advantage of a kinesiological law called 'reciprocal inhibition', in which your nervous system tells a muscle to let go of its contraction when the opposing muscle has work to do. In forward bends, contracting your quads facilitates the release of the hamstrings.

USING PROPS AND SUPPORT

As a rule of thumb, if your hamstrings are not yet flexible enough to allow your leg to stay fully extended in a forward movement, a solution may be to sit up with a folded blanket or firm cushion under your sitting bones to help tip your pelvis forward.

Keep your spine straight at all times. Never push yourselves in forward bends, either to overstretch the hamstrings or to the point of feeling pain in your sitting bones. To develop strong, stretch-tolerant hamstring tendons, start them with warming poses, including mild hamstring stretches such as Downward-facing Dog.

And, finally, a word about patience. The hamstrings are layered with lots of tough connective tissue – the gristly fibres that help hold the muscles' structure together. So you can't rush or hurry the hamstrings into flexibility; they need time to change their length – time in the sense that longer stretches, held with a belt (for 90 to 120 seconds), seem most effective with connective tissue.

CHAPTER 6

Meditation and the precious pearl

Meditation and de-stressing

In the centre of every stressful storm there is a place of total stillness: the 'eye'. In my life, I have found meditation to be one of the most powerful tools for creating this sense of peace within, even when the world around is in a state of tremendous flux or sometimes, even, chaos. Building a meditation cleanse practice is a bit like building a deposit account that you can withdraw from in times of need.

The yoga poses and intelligent movement described in Part 2 of this book are not techniques that are ends in themselves, but rather they culminate in meditation. This means we can sit in the meditative posture, with open hips, and our minds can remain undisturbed by the whims of the body. And through the 12-Day Plan our minds are energised and are less disturbed by toxic thoughts. We can enter into union.

You cannot control what happens outside yourself or what happens to you in life, but you can control your internal state of mind and how you react to negative things. How you respond to stressful situations is really the only thing that you do have control over. Worrying, getting angry and having arguments cannot change events that have already happened. They can only damage you by releasing stress hormones into your body, and the immune and digestive systems are those that suffer the most.

The breath is how you access your still and quiet self via meditation. By paying attention to the breath you bring the mind into the present moment in meditation, which is a wonderful thing because in it you find no worry and no suffering. So much of our time is spent in the future, worrying about careers and important life choices, perhaps, or spent in the past, going over negative events that have already happened, which we regret and feel that we could have done better with.

'In my life, I have found meditation to be one of the most powerful tools for creating this sense of peace within.'

WATER FROM A WELL

Meditation is like drawing water from a well. You build up the water levels in the well over time, and then when you need water you can draw it from the well. As you practise meditation you are contributing to the water levels of your well.

As part of the 12-Day Plan, I include a meditation to kickstart your day. This is a great way to become present in your own body and mind and your own life. You can tune in to what is best for you and connect with your gut feelings. Your gut can only benefit from the reduction in stress hormones (see page 70).

The flight-or-flight triggers in modern life have never been greater (see also page 72). While we rely on this rush of endorphins to get through hairy situations, remaining in a constant heightened state of alert is damaging to health.

The benefits of meditation

As you gain experience in meditation, you will gradually gain increased awareness of when you are either tense or relaxed, so that you can take steps to calm down when you begin to notice signs of stress. Through this awareness you will stop the release of harmful stress hormones that lower metabolism, energy levels, and even cause premature ageing.

'Stress is a huge factor in how your gut behaves, or misbehaves.'

The calming effect of meditation regulates the heart rate and blood pressure and facilitates the digestion and absorption of nutrients. Stress is a huge factor in how your gut behaves, or misbehaves, and at the root of stress is the fight-or-flight response – an adaptive reaction that through the ages served to protect us from emergency situations. The fight-or-flight response is controlled by stress hormones such as cortisol. If left unchecked, this response in the body can cause gut problems (as seen in Chapter 2), numbness, memory issues and insomnia. It is vitally important to counterbalance this response with relaxation – and meditation is perfect for bringing this about.

Meditation is an art that calms the soul and relaxes the mind, promoting an internal mental spaciousness in which troubles and fears no longer seem so menacing. Creative answers can naturally develop besides a confident detachment that provides better objectivity, perspective and the ability to concentrate.

Worrying and getting angry does not change the external events that have come about. In fact, they damage you by producing stress hormones and putting you in fight-or-flight mode, which puts your immune system and gut on high alert.

Meditation can take you out of that stressful state and into a state of peace, acceptance and gratitude.

It has also been demonstrated that meditation increases brain size. Researchers at Harvard, Yale and the Massachusetts Institute of Technology have found the first evidence that meditation can alter the physical structure of our brains and brain scans revealed that experienced meditators boasted increased thickness in parts of the brain that deal with attention and processing sensory input.

The structure of an adult brain can change in response to repeated practice of meditation. In one area of grey matter, the thickening turned out to be more pronounced in older than in younger people. Normally those sections of the human cortex become thinner as we age. The implication is that meditation may help slow some aspects of cognitive ageing. This is why Buddhist monks and yogis often enjoy an increased capacity for attention and memory in old age.

'Repeated thoughts and actions can rewire your brain.'

ALTERING BEHAVIOUR: NEUROPLASTICITY

Over the years, I have noticed that some of Mind Body Cleanse's most profound effects on health have to do with its ability to alter long-standing dysfunctional behaviours. People often have unhealthy habits of thought and deed that undermine their health; habits they may recognise but haven't been able to change so far. In addition to the direct health benefits of asana, pranayama, meditation and other yogic practices, it's not uncommon for regular practitioners to start eating better, to cut back on caffeine or alcohol, to quit jobs that make unreasonable demands on them, or to spend more time being in calming nature. Once people become more sensitive to the effects of different actions on their bodies and minds (whether it is [positively] practising alternate nostril breathing or [negatively] eating huge, fatty meals), they increasingly want to do what makes them feel better.

The modern understanding of the brain is that rather than being a static structure, this organ is constantly remodelling itself, a phenomenon scientists call 'neuroplasticity'. Repeated thoughts and actions can rewire your brain, and the more you do something the stronger those new neural networks become. Almost 2,000 years ago, Patanjali knew this when he suggested that the key to success in yoga is dedicated, uninterrupted practice over a long period of time. The resulting neural networks – or samskaras, as yogis call them – become stronger and stronger as you stick with the practice. Slowly but surely, these healthy grooves of thought and action help guide people out of the ruts in which they've been stuck, literally from lifetimes of accumulated karma.

'To understand
others is to have
knowledge;
To understand
oneself is to be
enlightened.
To conquer others
requires strength;
To conquer oneself is
even harder.'

LAO TZE

The precious pearl

Yogis and Taoists alike believe that every human is born with a precious pearl of original spirit deep inside the core of their being. As a human being matures from birth, this precious pearl gets buried deeper in the learned ignorance of education and socialisation. This pearl is undoubtedly our most unique human attribute and perhaps our only contact with the sacred. Sadly, many of us will go through life without ever realising it is there.

In the Himalaya, where I lived and studied for many years, I found yogic adepts transmuting essence and energy into pure spirit during meditation and pranayama. These adepts fasted frequently, controlled their diets strictly, often lived in complete solitude and spent entire days and nights meditating, strengthening their spirit-body.

'Meditation' is a poor translation of what the Masters simply call 'sitting still and doing nothing'. The real point of sitting still and doing nothing is to empty the mind entirely and to let the spirit endure in stillness and emptiness. Only in this meditative state will the spirit awaken fully and seek its unity with pure consciousness.

The final stage of meditation is only reached by a handful of advanced adepts, whose singular intention in cultivating physical health and longevity is to give themselves sufficient time and prana to prepare and complete the final stages of the internal alchemy that is required to create indestructible spirit-bodies.

These yogis form 'mysterious pearls', which grow with practice. These pearls form the embryo of the spirit-body. The spirit-body corresponds roughly in size and shape to the physical body, but it has no material substance. It is said that at the moment of death, the yogi enters into his spirit-body, eschewing the dissolution of consciousness and achieving spiritual immortality. Such adepts thus escape the endless cycle of birth and rebirth, as have the many avatars in human history.

Whereas Western dualism sees the spirit as independent of the body, yoga and Taoism regard the spirit as the flowering blossom of human life, with essence serving as its roots and energy serving as the connecting stem.

You do not have to be a nuclear physicist to realise that the strength of the integrity of the spirit are directly dependent upon adequate nutrition and ample energy. Only well-nourished roots planted in fertile soil generate strong stems and beautiful blossoms.

Tips for creating a happy mind

We can spend years listening to others tell us what's best for us, only to find that when we get our dream home, perfect body, bonus check or whatever it is we think we want, we still feel as if something is missing. Finding your purpose and passion in life isn't an overnight thing. But dedicating yourself to happiness, to practising the art of happiness, is a choice. When you commit to it, your entire life will transform.

Life, relationships and your career are full of ebbs and flows. And many of us are so busy trying to reach a goal, or get to some 'destination', that we forget to pause and enjoy the moments of excitement and awe along the way. In my life, I have had the good fortune (often coupled with dogged determination) to follow my heart. I haven't always been in the right place at the right time, but I would like to share with you the following practices that have helped me find true happiness:

Turn off the noise

It's important to turn off the 'noise' because all minds need a break! Learn to schedule time into your busy diary to switch off – you can literally call it 'switch-off time'. Turn off the TV, your phone and go back to the basics of a more simple existence. Light some candles, take a hot bath, bake chocolate brownies, read a new book, write things down. Create space and a time in your day to simply stop.

Morning practice

Each day I wake up with the gift of a clean slate and a chance to start afresh. How I begin my day has a huge impact on my mental and physical wellbeing, which goes to show that even the simplest habits can accumulate into huge health benefits over time. So, every day I start by reflecting on something positive that happened to me the day before. I am 'grateful' for the experience. I then take the positives and move forward. Being grateful creates powerful and positive emotions. My state of mind is immediately enhanced and I encourage positivity into my new day.

Train your mind

Learn to train your mind – otherwise your mind will control you. A detox such as the 12-Day Plan can be a period of glorious introspection and, as such, an ideal opportunity to learn how to start training your mind. Here's how. You can designate just two minutes per day to the preparation phase and then graduate to three, then five and so on.

- Find a comfortable place to sit, in a chair or on the floor
- Allow your natural breath to settle
- Bring your attention to your navel
- Observe the gentle expansion of your breath on the inhalation: observe the contraction of the breath back towards your spine on the exhalation
- Continue to observe the breath without forcing it
- When your mind wanders, as it inevitably will, bring it back to the breath
- Meditation occurs when the space between your thoughts increases.

Set your intentions for the Mind Body Cleanse

When you have experimented with meditation and would like to develop it further, you can try setting intentions. Intentions are the fuel to manifesting your goals and visions. Intentions help to create more clarity in your life, especially when the seed is planted right before you start your meditation.

An intention cannot be forced. It's a seed that you have to sow:

Here are four clear intentions to consider:

- I intend to be open to success and abundance
- I intend to forgive others, and myself
- I intend to make someone smile every day
- I intend to make meditation a more important part of my life.

Remember to keep the intention positive, uplifting and always in the present tense.

Make sure your intention can evolve, like a seed. If you stick with the same intention week after week, your mind will stop responding to it. The best way to resolve this is to make sure your intention or goal can easily be adjusted.

If your intention on your first day is to 'invite success and abundance into your life', after a few days you may change that intention to: 'My intention is to enjoy the success and abundance I create in myself.' Try not to alter your intentions dramatically or your goals too frequently. The aim is to polish and refine.

Aim your intention for the short term. You can still think of the big picture – just divide your long-term intention into a few shorter intentions instead. This will help you achieve an ambitious goal in shorter, more powerful, segments.

Once your intention is set, be sure to use it in your meditation. Start your meditation with a few deep breaths and observe the stillness within. Afterwards, bring your awareness to your heart and set your intention.

Stick to the same intention for a few days before moving on to the next one.

'Make sure your intention can evolve, like a seed.'

Keep talking to your body

A very important component of living a happy life is the nurturing and care of the physical body. Just as thoughts can affect us physically, the reverse is also true. For example, if you had a bad night's sleep, you might be tired and irritable. Without regular exercise and fresh air, your energy levels can drop and general motivation fade. So, practise an intelligent form of movement, such as yoga or Pilates, three times a week at least. Both yoga and Pilates are transformational, focused methods of movement that facilitate positive change in the body and mind.

List the things you are grateful for

To lift your morale and gain perspective, start to make a list of everything that you are grateful for in your life. It can be the simplest thing. Gratitude engenders positive thoughts and is a great way to get out of negative thinking. No matter how bad you feel, there is always something to be grateful for. For the next 12 days (of the 12-Day Plan) get into the practice of expressing daily gratitude and you will see that your life will change. Take stock and embrace the positive changes you are making.

Focus on changes you want to make

Avoid the mistake of only focusing on what's missing in your life. Instead, focus on the changes you want to bring about from a balanced and optimistic perspective. Remember to be realistic. Balance your drive for change with an appreciation of the here and now and your sense of disillusionment will go. If you are visual person, you can make a mood board of how you see yourself in wellness and optimal health. Pin up cuttings from magazines of things that inspire you. This will keep you motivated during the 12-Day Plan and once you have completed it.

Choose your words mindfully

Our words affect every action and thought we have, either positively or negatively. As our words can affect people around us, the same is true for their effect on us. Positively worded statements can create a positive mood and therefore a positive outcome. Choose your words wisely. The universe and your subconscious are listening and they will respond according to what they hear.

Love your imperfections

In today's society, we are constantly fed information telling us that we're not good enough just as we are. In the media, we're fed Photoshopped fairy tales in the form of an idealised appearances and lifestyles.

It has become clear throughout the quest to overcome my neck injury that I sustained in 2000 (see page 1), no matter how hard or often I practise, I am just not going to be able to bend my spine into certain positions that I used to pre-accident.

The miracle of this realisation is the recognition that my heart lives in this imperfect body. Embracing my body has helped me to learn how much pushing and striving is not only valuable, but it can also be highly destructive. Dwelling in my imperfect body has made me a more understanding teacher.

Forgive others, including yourself

The biggest shift for me came when I stopped looking at past mistakes as 'mistakes'. Instead, I realised how much I'd learned and grown as a result of each blunder. I forgave myself and realised that all is in perfect order.

Likewise, when you've crossed into adulthood, whether your childhood was happy or unhappy, understand that your parents just did their best for you with what they knew at the time. You will feel closer to them and accept them as they are. At the end of it all, it is love that matters most of all.

Love your sleep

Probably the most underrated of any of the issues listed here is sleep. Sleep is very important, so make sure that you are getting enough of it: lack of sleep is a modern malaise because people work long hours and then remain available 24/7 and this approach disturbs the body's delicate internal rhythms. A culture has also evolved that applauds those who exist on very little sleep – they have become focuses of our admiration because it is our perception that they work harder, are more dedicated and are somehow tougher because they 'need' less sleep. However, your mind and body gravitate towards predictability and the body becomes used to rhythms or routines. So stick with a daily routine and try to establish a regular sleep pattern: going to bed at the same time each night and getting up at the same time each morning. If you keep to a pattern, you are more likely to sleep well. Or practise some Pranayama (see below) that will engage with your rest and relaxation response.

Pranayama

Pranayama is the 'nutrition' provided by air through breathing and it is even more vital to our health and longevity than the nutrition provided by food and water via digestion. Breathing influences the body's bioelectric balance, just as diet influences its biochemical balance.

There are basically two functional types of breathing: cleansing and energising. Cleansing breath detoxifies the body and stresses exhalation, while energising breath collects and stores vital energy and focuses more on inhalation. Though people take breathing for granted, everyone unconsciously practises both types of breath spontaneously throughout the day, whenever toxins in the bloodstream reach a critical level or energy is running low. Thus, a sigh is a spontaneous cleansing breath, for it involves a quick inhalatory gulp followed by a long, forceful exhalation. By contrast, a yawn is a spontaneous, energising breath – a long, slow, deep inhalation, briefly retained in the lungs, followed by a relatively short exhalation.

Since breath and energy form a bridge between body and mind, breathing may be controlled either mentally or physically and is the only vital function that straddles the border of voluntary and involuntary control. Left unattended, breathing occurs as spontaneously and naturally as a heartbeat; when controlled by the mind, breathing becomes as deliberate as walking and can be made to regulate all other functions, including pulse, blood pressure, digestion, ejaculation, hormone secretion and so forth.

THE DIAPHRAGM AND THE BREATH

What distinguishes ordinary shallow breathing from deep abdominal breathing is the role played by the diaphragm. The diaphragm is a resilient yet flexible muscular membrane that separates the chest from the abdominal cavity. When the lungs expand, they push the diaphragm downwards; when they contract they pull it up into the chest cavity.

Though most Western physicians still regard the diaphragm as being a relatively unimportant muscle that is only passively involved in respiration, a cursory glance at nature reveals the fact that humans were meant to breathe primarily with the diaphragm, not with the ribcage and clavicles. Owing to laziness, ignorance and other factors, adults these days invariably become shallow chest-breathers rather than the deep abdominal breathers we were built to be. Chest-breathing employs the intercostal muscles between the ribs to forcibly expand the upper ribcage, thereby lowering air pressure in the chest so that air enters by suction. However, this leaves the lower lungs, which contain by far the greatest surface area, immobilised. Consequently, you need to take about three times as many chest-breaths in order to get the same quantity of air into the lungs as provided by a single diaphragmic breath.

'It is the most powerful muscle in our body; it acts like a perfect force-pump ... we have only to visualise the surface area of the diaphragm to accept the fact that it acts like another heart.'

Prana

The internal alchemy schools of Taoism that flourished during the early centuries AD thought of air as being the ultimate 'essence' of nature. Their aim was to purify their bodies and minds to the point that they could live on nothing but air and water, a diet they described as 'supping wind and sipping dew'. Prana, the vital energy contained in air, was literally regarded as a nutrient. While only the most advanced of adepts ever reach the goal of relying entirely on wind and water for sustenance, even the most ordinary of us can cultivate breath control as an effective means of promoting health and prolonging life. The act of breathing not only extracts prana from the air, it also drives and distributes prana through the body's invisible network of energy channels, or nadis. Nadis transport vital energy throughout the body and, when they get blocked, a condition called 'energy stagnation' occurs, resulting in insufficient blood circulation, which in turn causes such common ailments as lethargy, fatigue, weak libido and so on. Poor blood circulation and all its attendant ills can usually be remedied by correct breathing.

In the orient, breathing is regarded as a science. China has its chi-gung (meaning literally 'life energy cultivation'), which is a holistic system of coordinated body posture and movement, breathing and meditation used for health, spirituality and martial arts training, and India has pranayama, but the Western world lacks a specific term to denote breath control, nor do Western physicians understand how atmospheric energy serves as a vital 'nutrient' for human health. The implications for human health are manifold because understanding how the breath works and the importance of prana or life force are paramount.

'When correct breathing is practiced, the myriad ailments will not occur. When breathing is depressed or strained, all sorts of diseases will arise. Those who wish to nurture their lives must first learn the correct methods of controlling breath and balancing energy.'

DR SUN SSU-MO,
PRECIOUS RECIPES

Chi

Chi is the equivalent to the term 'prana' in the yogic tradition, taking many different forms within the human system. The most basic form is 'yuan-chi' or 'primordial energy'. This refers to the original burst of pure energy that occurs at conception and breathes life into the foetus in the womb. Yuan-chi can perhaps be compared to the potential energy that is stored in an ordinary battery. It begins to dissipate from the moment we are born and it determines our lifespan. One reason why children are so much more active and energetic than adults is that they have not yet polluted and dissipated their original primordial energy to the degree that adults have. That's also why children don't show as severe symptoms of poor diet and breathing as adults do; they are still protected by strong primordial batteries. But by drawing on these batteries to compensate for poor diet and other bad habits, they accelerate the rate of energy dissipation and sow the seeds of chronic debility in adulthood. Yuan-chi may be toned and enhanced though diet, herbs, proper breathing, sexual yoga and regular exercise.

Among the other forms of chi are:

- Yang-chi, which refers to vital energy in its volatile, kinetic and active form. It is the sort of energy that builds in the body during sexual intercourse and is absorbed directly from the atmosphere when breathing.

- Ying-chi is nourishing energy, which is extracted from the purest elements of digestion, from food and water.
- Wei-chi is protective energy, which is produced from the coarser byproducts of digestion. It circulates across the surface of the body, protecting the entire organism from invasion by extremes of the external environment.

When the chi of earth extracted from food and water meets with the chi of heaven absorbed from air, the two blend in the bloodstream to form the unique variety of vital energy that gives life to the human system. This is why diet and breathing are complementary approaches in cultivating health and longevity.

'The myriad ailments all begin with energy. The moment there is energy imbalance, any ailment might occur.'

YELLOW EMPEROR'S
CLASSIC OF MEDICINE

Despite its central role in yoga and other oriental philosophies, prana, or chi, remains the biggest stumbling block for Westerners studying mind-body cleansing techniques. Although Western scientists have no trouble dealing with radar, radio and gamma rays, ultraviolet light, electricity and other invisible forms of energy, they buck like wild horses when told that similar currents flow though and control the human system.

Since there is no equivalent term in English for 'chi' or 'prana', you can refer to it simply as 'bionic' or 'bioelectric' energy. This combines the idea of living energy uniquely associated with living organisms with that of electricity and negatively charged ions, which in scientific terms comprise the essential nature of chi or prana.

In the case of living organisms, the polarity of yin and yang and the tension that exists between them establishes the dynamic force field required to move chi, much as positive and negative polarity causes electric currents to move. The dynamics of ying and yang keep chi or prana in constant motion.

'(Chee) the vital force is the most subtle, most penetrating, most invisible agent we have known until now in nature. In this respect it surpasses even light, electricity and magnetism, with which in another respect it seems to have the greatest analogy.'

HUFELAND'S *THE ART OF PROLONGING LIFE*, 1838

In March 1968, the French newspaper *Le Monde* reported that the presence of negative ions in the air we breathe facilitates the absorption of oxygen and elimination of carbon dioxide in the alveoli of the lungs, whereas positive ions have the opposite effect. Toxic gases, dust, chemical fumes and so on all take the form of positive ions when released into the atmosphere, and these big spongy ions trap and absorb the light little negative ions, leaving the air virtually devoid of vitality. Pure country air contains an average ratio of two to three negative ions for every positive ion. In cities, the ratio drops drastically to one negative ion for every 300–600 positive ions.

Negative ions, prana or chi are thus the vital difference between pure and polluted air, not oxygen. A healthy body can purge itself of airborne toxins, but it can do absolutely nothing to compensate for a critical lack of prana in the air it breathes. The prime importance to human health and vitality of strong electric fields in the atmosphere is just beginning to be understood by Western science, although oriental mystics have realised it for thousands of years. So the lesson is clear, keep those bionic batteries fully charged at all times by breathing air that is full of vitality.

The air you breathe

In the early years of the space programme, scientists observed that astronauts became exhausted after just a few hours in their space capsules despite their robust health and physical fitness and it took decades to figure out why. The reason was the lack of good-quality air particles circulating in the enclosed space they inhabited.

Your office is not such a different environment. Good air – air that is full of vitality (or chi or prana) – is destroyed by air conditioning, central heating and closed windows. Working all day in air-conditioned or heated offices and factories often leaves us feeling totally drained, while farmers who spend the same number of hours outdoors doing strenuous physical labour do not suffer from the same feeling of depletion. It's not the work that is exhausting you by 6pm each evening, but rather the lack of vitality in the air you are breathing during the day. This explains why you feel refreshed after spending a day walking or mountain-biking in the countryside.

Just as correct diet enhances the body's store of nutrition, correct breathing of good quality air enhances the body's vitality and promotes blood circulation. Without this, lethargy, chronic fatigue, irritability, headaches, poor digestion and weak libido soon set in.

It is not the germs that make you ill – they are everywhere – it is the lack of resistance in your body because of toxins in the bloodstream that cause you to catch a virus. Having a low immune system opens a 'window of opportunity' in the body and permits germs to invade. In other words, germs are attracted to your internal condition. If you work in an office, the onset of the cold season can play havoc with your immune system and air conditioning merely circulates viruses among colleagues. But armed with a healthy, strong immune system you can keep the office flu at bay and avoid an energy slump during the winter months.

PART 2 The 12-day plan: taking action

CHAPTER 7

Overview of the plan

We can all benefit from doing the 12-Day Plan on a regular basis, at least quarterly, to chime with the changes that take place in every season. The plan can benefit young and old, first-time cleansers, performance athletes, those recovering from illness – and everyone in between. Typically spring and autumn are the best times, but summer is also good, and although perhaps not the best time to cleanse, winter can also work well. It's the best way to purge the body and is an essential tool in natural medicine because of its simplicity, low cost and therapeutic benefits. An effective cleanse will help you feel clear-headed and relaxed, experience easy digestion and regular bowel movements. With a fully functioning and healthy digestive system you can remain physically fit and mentally active for your entire life. You will sleep soundly and feel refreshed when you wake up – and, of course, you will experience weight loss.

If you carry out regular 12-Day Plans (3–4 per year) it can offer you the following. You can:
■ Eat a healthy cleansing, detoxifying diet
■ Be fitter and stronger, both physically and mentally
■ Lose weight – and keep it off
■ Have a clearer skin and sparkling eyes
■ Improve your gut health: digestion, assimilation of nutrients and elimination
■ Decrease or eliminate headaches, migraines, joint pain, body aches, colds and allergies and a whole list of minor health ailments
■ Increase your general motivation and enjoyment in life

- Make some positive lifestyle changes
- Concentrate better on anything you do and focus more easily
- Experience anti-ageing effects
- Live a 'greener' lifestyle.

For the Plan to be effective you must put aside at least three days of rest and relaxation for the main part of the total 12 days. This is how long it takes for the body's internal cleansing and healing mechanisms to shift into full gear. Seven days is even better because it takes all of that time of complete rest and clean living to start purifying the bloodstream and cleanse the internal organs and lymphatic system.

Remember to set a date to start the Plan (this helps you to fully commit to it). Make sure that you check ahead and look at your diary. Try to choose a period of relative calm in your life, such as a weekend, when you attempt the Plan and try not to embark on it when you have a busy period at work.

The Plan's cleansing and rejuvenating regime helps to accelerate the natural process of cleansing the system, purifying the body tissues and strengthening the immune system.

Fine-tuning your diet on the 12-Day Plan

The basic dietary strategy for an effective cleanse is to eliminate all acid-forming foods and beverages and imbibe only a few simple alkalising foods. What you *don't* eat is actually more important than what you *do* eat.

Foods to avoid

All processed foods, sugar, wheat, dairy, hydrogenated oils, carbonated soft drinks, coffee and alcohol, which contribute to the acidosis of the blood, must be excluded from your diet. If you are a coffee fiend try to reduce the amount of coffee you take in the days leading up to the 12-Day Plan.

Foods to choose

The food cornerstones of the 12-Day Plan are fresh fruits and vegetables. To make sure you have enough to choose from in your kitchen during the Plan stock up well in advance or order in – there are various organic box companies that deliver. The best-quality produce will be available at your local fruit and veg market/store/grocery or farmers' market.

The best vegetables to choose are the those that actively heal and cleanse the body, including sweet potatoes, yams, squash, pumpkin, carrot, beetroot, cabbage, asparagus, celery, parsley, spinach and all dark leafy greens. Feel free to include garlic and ginger in the 12-Day Plan in order to spice up the taste of your veggies.

You can prepare your vegetables in the following ways:
- Make a broth
- Steam, stew or stir-fry
- Drink freshly extracted raw vegetable juice.

A high vegetable content is recommended because of its ability to modulate liver detoxification. Also, vegetables contain a high level of soluble fibre, essential for rebuilding gut integrity. Chlorophyll in dark-green leafy vegetables, seaweed and wheat grass is particularly potent.
- Try to eat at least one helping of cruciferous vegetables daily. The cruciferous family, such as broccoli, kale, collards, Brussels sprouts and cauliflower, has the widest range of therapeutic benefits.
- Eat plenty of seasonal salad: lettuce, rocket, cucumber, celery, carrots, beetroot and olives. Add flavour using fresh herbs such as coriander, parsley, oregano, dill and basil. Dressings to go with your salad can include: cold-pressed organic extra-virgin olive oil, raw, unfiltered apple cider vinegar, lemon/lime juice and chopped garlic.
- Get your bioflavonoids from grapes, berries and citrus fruits.
- Eat organic food, if possible, to avoid accidentally taking petrochemical pesticides, herbicides, hormones and antibiotics.
- Eat beans, whole grains, fruits, nuts and seeds in limited quantities.
- Feed your gut with healthy bacteria – taking probiotics helps normalise gut flora and reduce endotoxins: toxins produced by imbalances in gut bacteria.
- Eat a few cloves of garlic every day.
- Try prepared herbal detoxification teas containing a mixture of burdock root, dandelion root, ginger root, liquorice root, sarsparilla root, cardamom seeds, cinnamon bark and other herbs. Decaffeinated green tea in the morning is also good.

Preparing your 12-Day Plan meals

'You can look forward to 12 days of delicious, nutritious, self-nurturing cuisine.'

There is no need to go hungry when you are doing the 12-Day Plan: in fact, you can look forward to 12 days of delicious, nutritious, self-nurturing cuisine.

■ **Buy foods that are really fresh.** Try to go organic or at least buy from a local farm shop or fresh fruit-and-vegetable supplier.

■ **Try to avoid ready-cut vegetables and fruit** because their nutritional value/enzyme integrity will be reduced before they get to you.

■ **Steam your fruit and veg.** Although some of the enzymes are destroyed through the heat, the moisture seals and preserves many of the active enzymes deep inside.

■ **Think about enzymes.** The presence of active enzymes is the distinguishing element between 'live' and 'dead' foods. These fragile compounds are easily destroyed by exposure to high heat, excess moisture, oxygen, radiation and synthetic chemicals that occur during cooking, canning, refining, preserving and pasteurising food. They are important biochemical catalysts secreted by the pancreas and other glands and organs, used for digesting food, metabolising nutrients and overall physical health.

■ **Try stir-frying.** While temperatures are high, cooking times are brief. The enzymes' integrity stays intact at the centre of the food.

■ **Eat raw food.** Foods brimming with enzymes are the most vital element for a healthy diet, and these can be found in raw fruit and vegetables.

■ **Aim to eat three meals a day** (apart from during the Power Phase, where all your food is liquidised).

SNACKS ARE IMPORTANT

When you miss meals or wait too long to eat, you may find that your body starts to hoard calories and fat. As a result, your concentration and energy may suffer and you might even start putting on weight. This means that when you do eat, you may end up over-eating, which strains the digestion and metabolism. So, be prepared, throughout your 12-Day Plan, with snacking ideas that will stoke your metabolic fires without overloading them. Each of us has different metabolic needs. While some of us thrive on a higher fat and protein diet, others need more of a balance. The best way to learn what is best for you is to listen to your body.

Some handy snack ideas:
> A handful of pumpkin seeds
> A small bowl of olives
> Hummus and a selection of raw vegetables for dipping
> A rice cake spread with unsalted hazelnut butter.

DO A KITCHEN DETOX

Being on the 12-Day Plan is a great time to do some household cleansing too – as well as your inner body. Cleanse both inside and out – and the kitchen is the perfect place to start. I do this every spring and autumn and get rid of all the kitchen items that are past their use-by date or that I do not need. Throwing out unwanted items makes you feel a lot lighter, both mentally and physically. It is difficult to have clarity when you live in a world of clutter. Ask yourself: what you do need and what you don't need – and be strict with yourself.

Go through your fridge/pantry/store cupboard and get rid of:
> All hydrogenated oils/trans fats
> Bottles that have gone past their use-by date – especially oils
> Sugar, high-fructose corn syrup, artificial sweeteners
> Anything with ingredients that you can't pronounce or those you are unfamiliar with – you won't be using it anytime soon
> Anything containing artificial colours or preservatives.

RECOMMENDED POTS AND PANS

Ceramic-coated non-stick

Porcelain-enamelled cast iron

Stainless steel

Bamboo products

KITCHEN UTENSILS AND STORAGE

Everyday items used in food storage and cookware often harbour health threats. Many of these engineered compounds bioaccumulate in our body's fat cells. In a recent study, an average of 200 industrial chemicals were found in the umbilical cords of ten newborns – notably stain and oil repellants used in fast-food packaging were discovered.

Think hard about what you are putting your food into. The Teflon chemical PFOA, found to be a causative toxin in the autism spectrum disorder, has been discovered in non-stick pans. Persistant organic pollutants (POPs) enter our bodies when we eat foods prepare on these surfaces. Over time these POPs slowly poison cellular energy, resulting in weight gain and fatigue. POPs have also been implicated in the worldwide explosion of diabetes and obesity.

FOOD STORAGE

Avoid plastic food storage containers that contain BPA or other bisphenols. Use containers made from glass or pyrex. Forgo clingfilm and instead use old-fashioned wax paper fastened with string or tape.

THE FOOD RULES FOR THE 12-DAY PLAN

Refer to this chart when you are planning your meals during the 12 days.

	YES	NO
Vegetables	All vegetables, including sweet potatoes and salad ingredients	Potatoes (apart from sweet potatoes)
Fruit	All fruit except those listed opposite	Mangoes, pineapples and bananas
Meat and fish	None	All fish, shellfish and meat
Nuts and seeds	Pumpkin, sesame, flax, sunflower seeds, and unsalted nuts such as hazelnut, Brazils, walnuts, almonds	Pistachios, peanuts, cashews
Pulses	Haricot beans, kidney beans, pinto beans, butter beans, chickpeas, lentils, lima beans	None
Grains and starches (make sure they are not processed or mixed with gluten-containing grains, additives or preservatives)	Amaranth, arrowroot, buckwheat, flax, gluten-free flours (rice, soy, corn, potato, bean), hominy (corn), coconut flour, millet, quinoa, brown rice, sorghum, soy flour, soy lecithin (pure), soy nuts (soaked soy beans, then air dried), soybeans, tapioca, teff	Cornflakes, rye flour, pasta, noodles, all bread, barley (malt, malt flavouring and malt vinegar are usually made from barley), triticale (a cross between wheat and rye), wheat*

* Avoiding wheat can be challenging because wheat products go under numerous names. Consider the many types of wheat flour on supermarket shelves – bromated, enriched, phosphated, plain and self-rising. Here are some other wheat products to avoid: bulgur, durum flour, farina, graham flour, kamut, semolina and spelt.

Oils	Extra-virgin cold pressed olive oil, pumpkin seed, borage oil, evening primrose oil, sesame oil, coconut oil	Sunflower oil, corn oil, avocado oil, canola oil, safflower oil
Dairy	None	All cow, goat and sheep produce – butter, cheese, cream, milk, yoghurt
Seasoning	Fresh and dried herbs, garlic, crumbled seaweed such as nori, dulse or kelp, ginger, chilli pepper, black pepper, cinnamon, curry, miso, tamari	Table salt, rock salt
Condiments	Raw unfiltered apple cider vinegar, lemon/lime juice	Mayonnaise, salad cream, tomato ketchup, brown sauce, soy sauce, vinegar
Drinks	Water, herbal teas, fruit teas, lemon in hot water	Coffee, alcohol, tea, soft drinks
Sweeteners	Honey, maple syrup, stevia. All taken in moderation	Sugar, artificial sweeteners, carob, corn syrup
Other	Mung beans, alfalfa sprouts, tofu, olives	Biscuits, cakes, eggs, margarine, canned foods, microwaved foods, processed foods

Drink plenty, but choose your drinks carefully
Water

In the West our drinking water is, surprisingly, far from clean and clear of toxins. Heavy metals have found their way into drinking water supplies, along with drug metabolites, such as antibiotics, sex hormones and mood stabilisers. Add to this the practice of chlorination to keep it free of bacteria, viruses and parasites and you have a harmful cocktail. Ingesting chlorine is not ideal for optimal health as it interferes with the functioning of the thyroid gland, which is the main driver of our metabolism.

Drink two to three litres per day of pure, preferably alkaline, water to flush away the large amounts of acids and other toxic wastes that the detoxing cleanse in the Plan process empties from the body.

Sipping hot water with lemon is a good idea and sage tea is excellent too.

How to improve your drinking water
Investing in one of these systems is an investment in your wellness and that of your family too.

- Carbon filters remove fluoride and chlorine from water, which gives it a cleaner taste.
- Distilled water benefits those undergoing a heavy metal detox. But, it is essential that trace minerals are replenished. This choice should only be made under the supervision of a health-care practitioner skilled in detoxification.
- Reverse osmosis systems remove drug metabolites, heavy metal ions and chlorine from tap water.

Juice
Raw juice retains all of the most active enzymes from the vegetables and can be made from any combination of the following: carrots, beetroot, broccoli, apples, celery, parsley, parsnips, coriander, parsley, ginger and wheat grass.

Drinking fresh juice helps to alkalise the system and is the most immediate and effective way to deliver vitamins, minerals and antioxidants straight into the body. It lies at the foundation of cleansing and acts to rebuild and rebalance your entire system. Aim for two to three glasses per day (300ml glass), apart for the Power Phase of the 12-Day Plan, where you may want to consume as much as six 300ml glasses per day. Remember to prepare your juice using fresh produce and drink it straight away.

Nearly all vegetables lend themselves to juicing, while some fruits are better juiced than others.

Lemon juice

Drinking a beverage with lemon in it first thing in the morning stimulates digestion and elimination. Lemon juice works wonders as a cleansing agent. It aids the liver in flushing out unwanted toxins, including those in the process of being absorbed into your body. It is high in vitamin C and a powerful antioxidant that boosts the immune system. As a superior alkaliser it also acts to purify the blood.

Nettle tea

Nettles have been used traditionally to treat rheumatism, eczema, arthritis, gout and anaemia. Surprisingly, although the nettle sting is highly irritating, once the leaves are dried and the acid is neutralised, they are a natural antihistamine. People tend to use nettles to treat urinary problems, urinary tract infections, kidney stones and allergies, or in compresses or creams for joint pain, sprains and strains.

Alcohol

During a cleanse, alcohol is a source of unnecessary calories and sugars and it is disruptive to sleep cycles, interacts with the neurotransmitter gamma-aminobutyric acid (GABA) receptors and blocks the brain's oxygen sensors. Therefore it is best to avoid drinking it altogether. The GABA receptors are a class of receptors that respond to the chief inhibitory compound in the central nervous system.

HOW TO MAKE NETTLE TEA
Use ½–1 tbsp of the dried herb and add to 1 litre of filtered water.

- Bring to the boil and simmer for 10 minutes
- Leave the tea to brew for 10 minutes
- Strain and put in a glass jar for the next day
- Drink at room temperature.

Caffeine

Caffeine interferes with the body's ability to absorb water and it quickly depletes the calcium and magnesium stores you need for bone health and for muscle contraction and relaxation. It is a powerful stimulant that blocks neurotransmitters for sleep and throws off the body's natural circadian rhythm. It also overworks our overused adrenals, which regulate stress. This is why I always advise clients who have difficulty sleeping not to drink coffee.

However, for many, giving up coffee can be a challenge. If you drink a lot normally, when you give it up you may experience some side effects, usually in the form of headaches. But you can prepare yourself in the days leading up to the 12-Day Plan. I always substitute every second coffee for a glass of water, so that by the time I start the Plan my withdrawal side effects are minimised.

Milk

Dairy products are a mucus-forming food, which in excess can clog your system. Research has shown that high bioavailable sources of calcium come from dark-green leafy vegetables, nuts and seeds. This research has also shown that magnesium, boron, vitamin D and vitamin K are as important to bone health as calcium. These minerals regulate the intake of calcium into the bone. Therefore, I advise you to get your calcium from vegetables and certain pulses rather than from a dairy source.

Your fruit and veggies
Fruits

The best choices of fruits are those that are semi-sweet originating from temperate climates. Examples are apples, pears, watermelons, black cherries and black grapes. Try to consume just one type of fruit at a time and 30 minutes either before or after your meal. Tropical fruits, such as mangos, pineapples and bananas, have a very high sugar content and tend to overheat the system, so it is best to avoid these. The exception is papaya.

Greens

It's important to consume greens while you are detoxing on the 12-Day Plan. You can take green supplements, such as my product 'Gorgeous Greens' (see also page 202), one of the supplements that I recommend taking during the 12-Day Plan, which contains:

- Organic spirulina
- Wheat grass
- Chlorella

- Alfalfa
- Kale
- Nettle leaf
- Dandelion leaf
- Ascophyllum nodosum
- Fucus vesiculosus.

'Gorgeous Greens' contains:

- Antioxidants that promote tissue healing/recovery
- Calcium, magnesium, potassium to regulate muscle contraction and relaxation
- Vitamins and minerals to boost energy and the immune system
- Seaweed to help regulate the metabolism naturally
- Dandelion leaf to help with digestion and the absorption of nutrients
- Anti-inflammatory qualities
- Electrolyte replacing qualities
- Natural fibre.

> **QUINOA**
>
> Quinoa is an alkaline and complete protein food. It is rich in amino acids, especially lysine, which is essential for tissue growth and repair. This high-protein grain also contains many minerals and B vitamins, and is an excellent alternative to rice.

Beans

- Wash beans or lentils in cold water. Soak lentils for one-and-a-half hours and beans overnight in three times the amount of water. Drain the beans and wash again before cooking.
- Eat beans or lentils unaccompanied by other proteins in the same meal.
- Try not to eat potatoes with beans, as potatoes will interfere with their digestion, and the room you are eating in will empty out quite quickly!
- Digestive spices, such as fennel and ginger, can help to make beans more digestible.
- Remember to chew your beans and start with easier types such as mung, adzuki and dal.

Herbs, spices and supplements

Herbs and spices possess potent nutritional benefits and all have their specific roles in the culinary realm. They can be used fresh or dried. The dried varieties tend to be more intensely flavoured and therefore they are often used in smaller quantities. You can grow fresh ones in beds or pots outside or on your kitchen windowsill inside.

Herbs

- Basil has anti-inflammatory and anti-bacterial properties and contains magnesium and betacarotene, which are good for the heart. Packed with antioxidants, basil can be used in tomato dishes, soups and salads.

- Bay is a natural antiseptic and protects the internal and external skin. It is rich in antioxidants betacarotene, vitamin C, zinc and selenium. Bay leaves are great in casseroles and vegetable dishes.

- Chives are known for their anti-bacterial, fungal and viral properties, and cleansing the gastrointestinal tract. They are part of the allium family and have superior levels of vitamins A and K, and are tart in flavour. You can use them in salads and soups.

- Coriander contains one of the highest levels of vitamin K as well as vitamins C and A: important for healthy bones, eye health and the gut. Coriander has microbial qualities and is good when used in Asian dishes.

- Mint helps ease digestion, stomach pain and bloating. It possesses gut-soothing, anti-bacterial and anti-microbial properties. You can use it to make a delicious tea, or with soups and salads.

- Parsley is packed with vitamin C, folic acid and flavonoids, which are all potent antioxidants that support heart health. It cleanses away bacteria in the mouth and is known to be the best natural toothpaste.

- Rosemary increases blood flow to the heart, head and brain, and its inflammatory properties help those with asthma and breathing difficulties. It is a pungent aromatic herb that stimulates the nervous system, creates alertness and concentration. It is delicious when used in a dressing.

- Sage creates anti-inflammatory responses in the bloodstream. It has stimulating effects on the neurons in the brain, aiding concentration and memory. It is tasty used in soups and casseroles.

- Tarragon increases bile production, which is good for making fats more digestible and providing antioxidants that support the gut function. It is also beneficial to heart health.

- Thyme helps to boost levels of DHA in the brain. It is a potent source of antioxidants and has abundant antimicrobial qualities. It is used in casseroles, soups and herbal teas.

ALOE VERA

The best way to take aloe vera is to use the purest concentration you can get hold of and add to freshly pressed juices and smoothies. My 'Hello Aloe' product (see page 203) is good for this. You can also add it to water.

Aloe vera:
> Offers anti-inflammatory, anti-spasmotic and cellular protective properties that benefit the gut.

It was used in many ancient civilisations and was touted as the 'miracle plant'.
> Is used as a tonic for a variety of ills including constipation, eliminating toxins and promoting digestion.
> May help to heal stomach ulcers and reduces the severity of stress-induced IBS. The inner-leaf-gel variety has been shown to have anti-bacterial properties.

CLEANSERS AND DETOXIFIERS

The following items helps to accelerate the natural processes of cleansing and detoxification in the body:
> Burdock, which can be found in my 'Super Absorb' product in the 2 Days programme (see page 202), has the ability to flush impurities from the body and it purifies the blood ('Super Absorb' is not sold seperately).
> The polyacetylenes in burdock inhibit the growth of bacteria and fungi, which prevents infections, especially skin infections.

> The inulin in burdock is a powerful immune system regulator. It attaches to the surface of the white blood cells to make them work better.
> Contains copper, iron magnesium, sulphur, biotin, zinc, iron, amino acids, and vitamins B1, B6, B12 and E.

DANDELION

I highly recommend using dandelion during your Cleanse. This can also be found in my 'Super Absorb' product (see page 000). It acts as a liver decongestant and restorative, liver gall-bladder stimulant, and as an antilipemic, an agent in the blood that reduces lipid levels.
> Gentle diuretic.
> Purifies the blood and liver and stimulates the manufacture of bile.

> Decreases the amount of serum cholesterol and uric acid.
> Optimises the performance of the kidneys, pancreas, spleen and stomach.
> Balances the hormones.
> Benefits the gut, balancing the enzymes that help digestion, assimilation and elimination.

Spices

- Cardamom helps combat infections by eliminating waste and toxins through the kidneys. It is excellent for digestion.
- Cinnamon has potent anti-inflammatory properties and is good for joint pain, IBS and skin problems. It regulates blood sugar by enhancing the effect of insulin.
- Chilli powder is great for heart health and improving cholesterol levels. Chillies are anti-bacterial, anti-fungal and help to lower blood-sugar levels. Chilli powder can also aid weight loss.
- Cloves help relieve indigestion and constipation and contain potassium for controlling blood pressure. They are also anti-inflammatory, anti-septic and anti-flatulent. They are packed with antioxidants, vitamin A, betacarotene, omega-3 fatty acids and vitamins.
- Fenugreek can be used as a laxative, digestive and a remedy for coughs and bronchitis. The seeds are high in soluble fibre, which helps to lower blood sugar, making them key in improving the symptoms of diabetes. It is also used to help reduce irritability during menopause and PMS.
- Ginger soothes the respiratory tract and helps common colds and coughs. This warm spice also helps reduce arthritic, joint and muscle pain while aiding digestion.
- Juniper is high in antioxidants and has the ability to improve your digestion as bitters cause saliva, digestive enzymes and stomach acid to increase.
- Nutmeg stimulates the brain, improves concentration, helps soothe stress, fatigue, anxiety and depression, and can be used to relieve painful aching joints and muscles. It also helps to relieve digestive problems and is used to improve sleep. Nutmeg contains potassium, calcium, iron, magnesium and zinc.
- Turmeric improves liver detoxification and supports the immune, digestive and nervous systems. It provides potent antibacterial, antiviral and antifungal properties. It is also used to treat wounds and skin conditions such as psoriasis.
- Vanilla is a great source of antioxidants and has anti-inflammatory and anti-bacterial properties. This spice also has a calming effect, which can help to relieve anxiety.

L-glutamine

This is one of the most abundant amino acids in the body and the preferred source of energy for the cells that line the small intestine. The best way to take it is to dissolve 1 gram of powder in water or added to freshly pressed juices and smoothies on an empty stomach. For best delivery to the electrolytes, the powder form is best. L-glutamine taken between meals can also help curb sugar cravings. It:

- Minimises the breakdown of muscle tissue and improves protein metabolism for use after exercise.
- Can also be used first thing in the morning to help rebuild the lining of the digestive system. This helps to maintain the gut barrier function.
- Provides fuel for the immune system and can assist the healing process after surgery.

Vitamin D3

There is a great deal of research available on the importance of this vitamin, especially at sun-limited times of year. Vitamin D3, as found in my product 'Magical Multi' (see page 203) is essential for promoting calcium absorption in the gut. Vitamin D has other roles for our health including modulation of neuromuscular and immune function and reduction of inflammation.

Vitamin D has been found to:
- Strengthen bones
- Strengthen the immune function
- Reduce tumour growth
- Reduce cancer risk
- Reduce risk of multiple sclerosis
- Lower risk of diabetes
- Decrease symptoms of seasonal depression.

Vitamin B complex

Improves energy levels, nerve conduction and concentration. Since vitamin B levels in the body are reduced by stress, caffeine and alcohol, this is another supplement that I recommend for general health.

TRY SOME FERMENTED FOODS

Central Europeans have long eaten pickled and fermented foods, as have the Japanese. For Koreans, kimchi, or pickled cabbage, is the national dish. Fermented foods provide health benefits through the way in which the inherent bacteria, yeasts and moulds predigest foods and create probiotics that introduce bacteria to the gut.

Fermented vegetables have an alkaline effect once they have been digested. It is their role in stimulating the hydrochloric acid in the stomach that is so important. Stress interferes with the stomach's production of hydrochloric acid, which shuts down the 'rest and relaxation' response. In a highly stressed situation, digestion is put on hold. This has a knock-on effect because whatever is not working at the top end of the gut will affect the other parts of the gut too.

Sauerkraut is made by cutting and crushing raw vegetables to release the fluids they contain, then layering them with salt to create a fermentation that breaks the vegetables down into a more easily digestible product. Traditional sauerkraut uses cabbage as a base.

Some nutritional tips for life

The basic dietary strategy for long-term health is to eliminate all acid-forming foods and beverages and consume only a few simple alkalising foods that require the least energy to digest. Here are some useful tips to add to the mix.

- Increase your consumption of fresh, locally grown fruit and vegetables in season, preferably organic.
- Make sure that you consume fruit and vegetables as close to their natural raw state as possible. If you have to cook them, then steam or stir-fry briefly.
- Increase your intake of water to up to two to three litres per day.
- Do not eat after 8pm at night.
- Stop eating when you are 70 per cent full. If you are still hungry 30 minutes later, then eat some more.
- If you find yourself craving carbohydrates and sugar, have a snack of protein and fat, then wait 30 minutes. Protein and fat are much more satisfying than carbs and sugar.
- Don't count your calories.

Try to:

- Switch cakes, biscuits and crisps for dried fruit, seeds and unsalted nuts such as pumpkin, sesame, flax, sunflower, pecan, hazelnuts and Brazils. Pistachio and cashew nuts are okay in between 12-Day Plans.

Swap white bread, rice and pasta for their brown, organic equivalent, but restrict the servings to one per day. If you are gluten-intolerant make sure that you eat a suitable gluten-free alternative.

- Ideally eat three servings per week of pulses and beans such as lentils, chickpeas, haricot, aduki and butter beans.
- Limit the quantity of animal protein in your diet to two servings per week, or certainly no more than 10 per cent of your diet, and choose organic or grass-fed meat where possible. Focus on reducing your intake of red meat (beef, lamb, pork) as well as smoked meats such as salami. Consider having fish, chicken or vegetarian alternatives such as tofu.
- Ideally have two servings per week of oily fish such as salmon, sardines and tuna. Avoid salmon and tuna if you are pregnant.
- Reduce your intake of coffee. Start by having water instead of every second cup of tea or coffee.
- Reduce your intake of carbohydrates such as potatoes and pasta.
- Reduce your intake of refined sugar and consider having honey or maple syrup instead. Try reducing, then eliminating, sugar from food and drinks. It is surprising how quickly you can get used to less-sweet things.
- Use only unrefined oils such as cold-pressed virgin olive oil. Avoid hydrogenated fats.
- Reduce your intake of salt. Try to flavour food with seaweed (nori or kelp), tamari or shoyu sauce, fresh and dried herbs.
- Avoid chemical additives and preservatives – remember to read the label.

Using yoga in the 12–Day Plan

A daily yoga asana and pranayama practice is a must during the 12-Day Plan. Yoga can aid the body in the detoxification process by encouraging lymph drainage and increasing blood flow, thus facilitating the elimination of metabolic toxins through the excretory pathways of the body such as the liver, kidney, skin and lungs. Practise yoga in conjunction with slow, deep, rhythmic breathing that fully engages the diaphragm. The combination of slow stretching and loosening the limbs drives blood and lymph through the body like a strong pump.

I recommend a combination of twists, backbends, forward bends and supported shoulder stands and inversions, which help to drain lymph

QUICK-REFERENCE YOGA CHART

PREPARATION PHASE

 1 Sun Salutation (see page 128 for complete sequence)

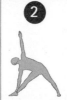 **2**

 3

 4

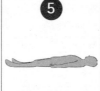 **5**

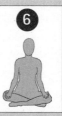 **6**

PRE-PURIFICATION PHASE

 1 Sun Salutation (see page 128 for complete sequence)

 2

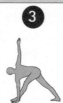 **3**

 4

 5

 6

 7

POWER PHASE

 1 Sun Salutation (see page 128 for complete sequence)

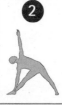 **2**

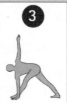 **3**

 4

 5

 6

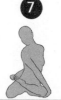 **7**

MAINTENANCE PHASE

 1 Sun Salutation (see page 128 for complete sequence)

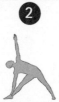 **2**

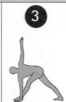 **3**

 4

 5

 6

 7

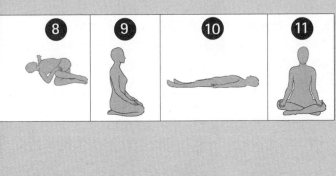

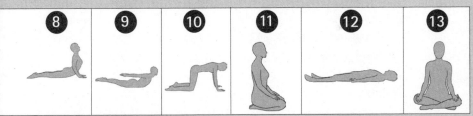

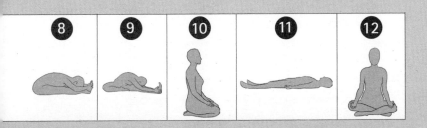

from the legs. Twists increase peristalsis, clear stagnation, increase agni (digestive fire) and help to send blood through the liver. Support your asana practice with energising pranayama practices such as Kapalabhati (see page 133). Deep diaphragmatic breathing saturates the bloodstream with fresh supplies of oxygen, while purging it of carbon dioxide, thus accelerating the cleansing process.

In this chart you will see how to use intelligent movement in your 12-Day Plan and you will see how the practice builds systematically from one phase of the Plan to the next. Preparation Phase is just that – a gentle warm-up for your body and mind. In the Pre-Purification Phase I add in some twists. In the Power Phase I add bends and inversions too. And then in the Maintenance Phase I add in forward bends too. In addition, I will be guiding you through some pranayama techniques and meditations. You will see that a numbering system **0**, both on the Quick-Reference Yoga Chart and in the text, helps you work through your exercises in the right order.

Take a holistic approach

Cleansing is a journey from the old you to the brand-new you. It is a great opportunity to start taking a more holistic approach to your health and wellbeing. Take the opportunity of doing the 12-Day Plan to try out some new things to support you, if you wish (though they are optional and not shown on the chart as part of the Plan – add them as and when you like):

Massage

The deep pressure of massage stimulates various vital points along the bioelectric network (in yoga we refer to these vital points as 'nadis') and dislodges toxic deposits in the tissues. The massaging action scatters the released toxins and facilitates their drainage through the blood and nymph. Always drink at least one or two large glasses of pure alkaline water immediately after a therapeutic massage.

Rolfing

Rolfing is a deeper massage that works on the fascia, or connective tissue, that surrounds the muscle. Rolfing can access deeper core muscle, such as the diaphragm.

Acupressure
Like acupuncture, acupressure works with the bioelectric energy flowing through the meridian energetic network in the body. Instead of using needles (as in acupuncture), pressure is applied using the elbows, feet and hands. If you would rather avoid needles, this method might be worth trying.

Walking and swimming
Try fitting in 20 minutes of walking per day into your usual routine. Build this up to 45 minutes. You can take this in the form of three 15-minute walks if that works better with your schedule. Swimming is also excellent. Not only will the exercise do you good but the fresh air will make you feel invigorated (see also page 93).

Detoxifying meditation
Meditation helps to bring a balance of mind, body and spirit, which aids the process of detoxification of both the mind and body. Cleansing the mind of negative thought patterns is essential to detoxification. Becoming more conscious of these patterns will add new depth to the cleansing process. True detoxification is multifaceted; it means not just isolating the body but also taking your mental and emotional state into account.

Three-Month Breathing Practice
The Mind Body Cleanse sequences in this book can help you to quiet your mind so you can feel, and then release, the tension stored in your gut and other places in your body. These unconscious tensions, which can become knots along the abdominal muscles or a restricted diaphragm prevents you from taking full, deep breaths. This can perpetuate gut issues and other body-wide health problems.

I prescribe the following Three-Month Breathing Course for anyone who has gut problems, such as IBS, or has difficulty digesting food. The breathing practices are best done daily at the same time of day, preferably 30 minutes before you eat.

Month 1/Breathing Practice 1
Three-part breath and complete breath
Sit in a comfortable cross-legged or kneeling position. If you are sitting, place a yoga block under your behind so that you are half on and half off it.

Sectional breathing: each day you work through the whole sequence. Allow your natural breath to settle before you start.

A Visualise the air flowing into your abdomen	x12
B Visualise the air flowing into your ribs	x12
C Into the top lobes of your lungs	x6
D Complete yoga breath	x12

Alternate the method of filling and emptying the lungs – whichever feels more comfortable for you.

Month 2/Breathing Practice 2

Sectional breathing: each day you work through the whole sequence. Allow your natural breath to settle before you start.

	Inhale	Exhale	
A Visualise the air flowing into the abdomen	1	1 ½	x6
B Visualise the air flowing into the ribs	1	1 ½	x6
C Into top lobes of lungs			x6
D Complete Hatha yoga breath	1	1 ½	x12

Alternate the method of filling and emptying the lungs – whichever feels more comfortable for you.

Month 3/Breathing Practice 3

Ratio breathing – extending the breath with complete Hatha yoga breath. Allow your natural breath to settle before you start.

Inhale	Exhale	
1	1	x3
1	1 ½	x3
1	2	x6
1	1 ½	x3
1	1	x3

Relax hands
Natural breath

Skin-brushing

The skin is the largest organ in the human body and skin-brushing assists the lymph system to cleanse itself of the toxins that collect below the skin. Brush the skin for three to five minutes daily, in the mornings, on dry skin, before you wash. Use a natural fibre brush with a long handle – remember to skin-brush towards the heart.

Tapping

Tapping is a great pick-me-up for increasing focus and rejuvenating the body and mind. You can tap on your face, head, neck, shoulders, chest, abdomen and lower back to boost the immune system by increasing production of T-cells. The technique also reduces stress, energises, increases focus, promotes strength and vitality, and balances the left and right hemispheres of the body. The healing concepts that tapping is based on have been used as part of Eastern medicine for over 5,000 years. Like acupuncture and acupressure, tapping is a set of techniques that utilise the body's energy meridian points. You can stimulate these points by tapping on them with your fingertips – literally tapping in to your body's own energy and healing power.

The basic technique requires you to focus on the negative emotion at hand: a fear or anxiety, a bad memory, an unresolved problem or anything that's bothering you. While maintaining your mental focus on this issue, use your fingertips to tap between five and seven times each on 12 of the body's meridian points. Tapping on these points while concentrating on accepting and resolving the negative emotion will access your body's energy, restoring it to a balanced state.

Progressive muscular relaxation

The main aim of progressive muscular relaxation is to allow you to feel the difference between tense and relaxed muscles. You recognise when your muscles are tense, and then, in response, you relax them. The technique involves tensing the muscles as hard as you can while concentrating on the sensation you feel in them. Hold the tensing action for a few seconds and then experience the difference in how they feel when they are relaxed. The progressive muscular relaxation process involves going through all parts of your body, starting with the feet, and it's best to practise with a teacher first of all so that you can get the hang of it.

Step-by-step technique

1. Pull your toes back, tense the muscles in your feet and relax.
2. Straighten your legs, push your heels away, tense your whole leg and repeat.

3. Arch your back, relax and repeat.
4. Tense your stomach muscles by pulling them in, relax and repeat.
5. Clench your fists, tense and tighten. Feel your whole arm tighten hard enough through all the muscles to your shoulder.
6. Shrug your shoulders up to your ears as hard as possible, bringing them up and in. Shuffle them back down, lengthening the back of your neck.
7. Screw up your face several times and then relax.
8. Tense your whole body and then relax.

You can now go through the body again, emphasising any tense areas that you are still aware of.

Autogenic relaxation techniques
Use your mind to relax your physical body. Isolate and relax in turn (as you did for Progressive muscular relaxation) all the muscles in your body, but without tensing the muscles first. This technique is very effective for IBS.

Visualisation techniques
Visualisation techniques are also great for relaxation. This technique is perfect if you are a visual person: it involves focusing on a colour, such as green. Picture a meadow and its freshness, the young green grass. Breathe into the colour and let it fill your eyes, the space in front of your eyes and the space behind them. Finally let your whole body fill with green.

You can also focus on a flower, which you place in front of you at a comfortable distance. Your aim is to touch and smell the flower and examine it in its entirety. Allow the flower to become soft focus and then close your eyes and visualise it in your head. Gradually let the flower go and become aware of the breath.

Positive affirmation
'How am I right now?' 'Am I feeling fine?'

With positive affirmation you listen to your body rather than your mind. This technique is like clearing a space in a cluttered room and is most effective for consulting your own inner wisdom. It involves turning your attention inwards, to your 'felt sense' of a particular problem or situation. If you use it successfully it identifies and localises your most important problem and your existing hidden knowledge of it. This ultimately brings a shift in your felt sense of the problem, and relief and insight about what practical steps you can take next. This technique has the advantage of creating distance from whatever it is you are concerned about or the problem, while acknowledging that these things exist and are yours.

Using positive affirmations is easy to do yourself, but generally it is better if you are led through the technique by a competent teacher, either in a class or via a recording, so that you can hear the instructions and follow them uninterrupted. You will be asked to repeat the positive affirmation a number of times.

Steaming

Steam and heat help to promote the excretion of toxins through the skin. If you do not have access to a steam room, take a hot bath, add some of your favourite essential oil or mineral salts, lie back and relax.

Regular infrared sauna therapy use provides an excellent natural health pathway to improving heart health. A study from the February 2011 issue of *Circulation Journal* shows just how positively the heart responds to infrared sauna. In the study, researchers from the Department of Cardiovascular, Respiratory and Metabolic Medicine, Kagoshima University, Japan, showed that oxidative stress in heart patients is remarkably reduced with repeated daily infrared saunas.

Essential oils and baths

Indulge in Himalayan rock salt, and add some detoxifying essential oils at any phase during your 12-Day Plan. Or you can use 'Buddhi Bath'. Pour the entire contents of the sachet (see page 203). Lie back and relax! Remember to get out of the bath slowly.

Epsom salts are an ancient remedy for drawing out toxins. Taking one or two of these baths every week will help to encourage weight loss. Add one or two mugs of Epsom salts into a hot bath.

GENERAL GUIDELINES FOR A GREENER LIFESTYLE

Try some (or all) of the following guidelines to help you adopt a really green lifestyle.

> Drink filtered water (reverse osmosis or carbon filter)
> HEPA/ULPA filters and ionisers can be helpful in reducing dust, moulds, volatile organic compounds and other sources of indoor air pollution
> Clean and monitor heating systems to detect the release of carbon monoxide
> Keep houseplants around your home to help filter the air
> Air out your dry-cleaning before you wear it
> Avoid excess exposure to environmental petrochemicals (garden chemicals, car exhaust)
> Reduce or eliminate the use of toxic household and personal-care products (aluminium-containing underarm deodorant, antacids, and pots and pans)
> Remove allergens and dust from your home as much as possible
> Minimise electromagnetic radiation (EMR) from radios, TVs and microwave ovens
> Reduce ionising radiation (from sun exposure or medical tests such as X-rays)
> Reduce heavy-metal exposure (lead paint, thimerosal-containing products, etc.)
> Have 1–2 bowel movements a day
> Drink 6–8 glasses of water a day
> Work up a sweat regularly by doing brisk exercise, by walking briskly, swimming or cycling.

THE FOUR PHASES OF THE 12-DAY PLAN

The 12-Day Plan is devised in order to approach cleansing in a systematic way over the course of the 12 days.

Days 1–3/Preparation Phase. This part of the 12-Day Plan is very easy indeed. Eliminate all of the 'no' foods and introduce foods from the 'yes' section in The Food Rules (see chart, page 100).

Days 4–6/Pre-Purification Phase. Now you start to streamline your diet in order to condition your body for optimum cleansing during the Power Phase, which comes next. Eat as much raw food as possible, especially if you are doing the Cleanse during the warmer months of the year. Otherwise there are some delicious soup recipes (see page 177), which are ideal for winter.

Days 7–9/Power Phase. You should be feeling pretty good by now, having spent the last six days absorbing the nutrients from simple, healthy foods. By consuming nothing but liquids and giving your digestion a break, consuming raw, fresh juices and smoothies for the three days of the Power Phase, you give your body a break from normal food and drink. This gives your system the chance to do its own bit of housework, gobbling up unwanted microbes, toxins and matter, to leave you feeling rejuvenated.

Even though this part of the 12-Day Plan is where you will be taking liquids only, you should not feel hungry.

Days 10–12/Maintenance Phase. Well done! You have completed the Power Phase, eliminating a vast amount of toxic waste from your body and giving your digestive system a full service. (continued)

(continued)

For most people, following a cleanse plan will be perhaps the most powerfully purifying endeavour of their life and be a truly life-changing experience. On a physical level, when the blood and tissues of the body have been purged of poisons, degeneration is arrested and germs are given a smaller window of opportunity to attack – the body's natural healing mechanisms repair the damage and restore optimal health to the whole system. The effects on other levels of our being are even more profound. Our mental faculties generally improve. Emotionally we are able to let go of baggage as we let go of its physical counterpart. Our energetic levels change and we encourage and attract greater positivity into our lives.

How often should I do the 12–Day Plan?

Carrying out three or four 12-Day Plans a year is recommended, while you take care of your diet, by eating healthily, in between times. Almost anyone is capable of completing a 12-day fast, but if you have never tried it, you might want to experiment with a few 3-day mini-fasts first as a warm-up. A mini-fast is a good way of working your way up to a full 12-Day Plan, as well as being an excellent form of maintenance between longer therapeutic fasts. For a 3-day fast you can follow the dietary guidelines on page 100–10. The '3R' 3-day cleanse product (see page 202) is a gentle and condensed cleanse lasting three days which contains all the ingredients that you need to complete a gentle and effective cleanse. It will also help to 'mend' your gut.

In addition to doing four 12-Day Plans every year, I fast for one day every week, taking nothing but pure alkaline water, or if I wish, juices or smoothies. This gives my digestive system a rest and allows my body a brief break in order to restore and rejuvenate it.

After the 12–Day Plan

After the 12-Day Plan it is good to revisit all your priorities and goals and make plans for the future. The best part about trying out the different techniques in this book is that, as you move forwards after the 12-Day Plan, you will understand the effect of each technique and when and how to use it. You will come to a better understanding of what nourishes your body and what pollutes it, and, as a result, you have the tools to put together your own cleanse plan and personalise it to your own needs.

LOTS of fresh fruit and vegetables

Herbal teas

Nuts, seeds, pulses

A juicer for vegetable- and fruit-juicing

Water filter

Natural fibre brush for skin-brushing

A journal

Getting started

Preparation is the key to a successful cleanse.

First of all, take 20 or 30 minutes to draw up a list of things you may need to buy. You will be consuming plenty of fresh fruit and vegetables (see The Food Rules chart, page 100), herbal teas and nuts, seeds and pulses. Acquire a juicer for vegetable- and fruit-juicing (it needn't be an expensive one) and get hold of a water filter if you don't already use one.

Buy a natural fibre brush for skin-brushing and also a journal to write in. It is a good idea to record your thoughts and feelings, any changes, improvements and psychological effects you may experience. You can also write down any positive affirmations. If you decide to eat out during the 12-Day Plan, try to choose dishes that are nutritious and Cleanse-friendly and try to stay focused – don't be tempted to lapse and think that you'll get back on track again tomorrow because consistency is important in achieving good results.

Try to plan your 12-Day Plan so that you go through the Power Phase during a period of relative calm – time off work or a quiet time when you don't have any demanding commitments or distractions are ideal.

TIPS TO GET YOU THROUGH

Here are a few last-minute words of advice before you start on the Plan.

> If you are a coffee fiend, try to reduce the amount you take in the days leading up to your start date.
> Replace every second cup with a glass of water.
> Refer to The Food Rules list on page 100.
> Making time for relaxation is very important. Try to plan the 12-Day Plan so that you do the Power Phase (Days 7–9) in a period of relative calm. A weekend or a quieter patch at work would be ideal.
> You will also need to make an appointment with your local colonic hydrotherapist if you are congested or suffer from constipation. However, I appreciate that colonic hydrotherapy might not be to everyone's liking.
> Try to stay focused on the Plan – don't lapse.

RECORDING YOUR PROGRESS DURING THE 12-DAY PLAN

You can record, in diary form, the effects (physical, mental, emotional or spiritual) of your personal practice. Over time you will notice how that particular practice affects you. Try out the diary layout suggestion below and, when you notice something different, good or not so good, make a note. You do not need to write something down every day, just when you observe a change.

NAME:

Date / time	Practice	Comments

CHAPTER 8

Preparation phase/days 1–3

Today you will start a daily practice of Sun Salutations, breathing practice and meditation that you will continue to do throughout the 12-Day Plan. The Sun Salutation stimulates the entire musculoskeletal system as well as many of the internal organs and is a great way of starting the day as you mean to go on. See the chart on page 112 to show you how the regime of yoga asanas gradually builds up over the 12 days of the Plan.

Your checklist

- Follow the nutritional guidelines (see pages 137–43) and try out some of the suggested recipes
- Drink hot lemon water first thing in the morning
- Do your Mind Body Cleanse Practice (see below)
- Try skin-brushing
- Drink freshly squeezed juices
- Drink plenty of water
- Make sure you've booked your colonic hydrotherapy sessions for the Power Phase – if you need it
- Start using your journal to record thoughts and feelings.

MIND BODY CLEANSE PRACTICE/THE PREPARATION PHASE

PREPARATION PHASE

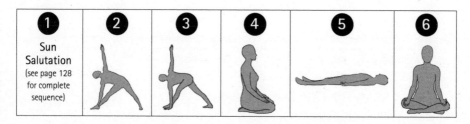

1 Sun Salutation (see page 128 for complete sequence)   **2**   **3**   **4**   **5**   **6**

Before practice

When you do your yoga practice first thing in the morning, make sure that you practise on an empty stomach – especially before the twisting poses (see pages 130–3). If you usually feel hungry on waking up, take liquid nutrients such as a high-quality greens powder ('Gorgeous Greens', see page 104), or something small and light without too much fat or protein, which can slow digestion.

I like to have a greens powder drink ('Georgeous Greens') before an early morning practice and a smoothie afterwards. If my yoga session is later in the morning I tend to have a smoothie beforehand.

If you are doing yoga later in the day, eat full meals two to four hours before your practice. This time will vary from person to person, but your practice should not interfere with the digestive process. For people with a speedier metabolism, have a small snack, such as some nuts or a piece of fruit, an hour before yoga to provide you with a steady source of energy fuel.

After practice

Within an hour of your yoga session, take a good source of protein along with vegetables to replace vital minerals, rebuild muscle and stoke the metabolic fire.

Ujjayi technique

Try Ujjayi (or 'victorious') breathing whenever you practise yoga asanas. You will find it both energising and relaxing. This style of breathing calms the heart and mind and soothes the nervous system. The Ujjayi pranayama technique also stimulates the vagus nerve, which triggers your nervous system into rest-and-relaxation mode. This is why Ujjayi is a great technique to use if you are feeling stressed and it is very useful if you suffer from IBS-related disorders.

■ The sound of Ujjayi breathing is created when you gently constrict the opening of your throat to create some resistance to the passage of air. If you gently pull your breath in on inhalation and gently push it out on exhalation against this resistance you can create a well-modulated and soothing texture to your breath, like the sound of ocean waves rolling in and out.

- Try to find a brief pause at the top of the inhalation and at the end of the exhalation. This will let you feel patience in your breath and allow your mind to ride on its surface.

- It is important to remember that the key to Ujjayi breathing is relaxation and the action of Ujjayi naturally lengthens your breath. You will need to make a small effort to produce sound, though too much effort creates a grasping quality and a grating sound. Generally, you will find the inhalation more challenging, so begin by practising on the exhalation, where there is a natural letting-go.

- To practise the inhalation, focus on creating a soothing and pleasing sound that feels unhurried and unforced. Work on your Ujjayi breathing sitting in a relaxed cross-legged position. Imagine sipping the breath in through a straw. If the suction is too strong the straw collapses and you will need to use great force to suck anything through it. Once you master Ujjayi breathing while sitting, the challenge is to maintain the same quality of breathing throughout your asana practice.

- Try to maintain the length and smoothness of the breath as much as possible. Once you find a baseline Ujjayi breath in a pose that is not too strenuous, try to maintain that quality of breath throughout the practice. Some asanas require great effort and you may begin to strain in your breathing. This means you may be pushing yourself too hard. Use that feedback as a guide; if you start to strain, it may be time to come out of the pose and rest.

- Practising Ujjayi breathing is a way of harnessing the mind and body, using the breath as a vehicle for taking attention off your normal thought patterns and refocusing it on the physical details of practice.

- The breath has a purpose on the physical level as well; you can stretch more deeply into the poses and, as you begin to move more and the practice becomes more rigorous, it becomes harder to maintain a steady, even Ujjayi breath. You may start to breathe through your mouth and your breath may become shallower and more ragged.

- Maintaining a steady Ujjayi breath is hard work but it has great benefits – enhancing the purification and nourishment of each and every cell and having a positive effect upon your lungs and heart, as your breath will naturally become deeper and faster with increased effort.

THE GENTLE BREATH

Ujjayi breath is very gentle.

It is not necessary to breathe loudly or aggressively. Ideally, the Ujjayi breath is soft in nature and volume. While the sound will be audible to someone close by, it's not necessary for the sound to fill the whole room! The quality of the Ujjayi breath is not measured in volume, but in length and steadiness. Rather, bring your awareness to the constancy that this breath gives you. Evenness of breath will give you evenness of temperament.

Ujjayi breathing: step-by-step

Start with 5–8 minutes of practice. Gradually increase to 10–15 minutes.

1. Inhale through your nose, then exhale slowly, mouth wide-open. Direct the outgoing breath slowly across the back of your throat with a long 'ha' sound. Repeat several times, then close your mouth.
2. Now, as you both inhale and exhale through your nose, direct your breath again slowly across the back of your throat. Ideally, this will create, and you should hear, a soft hissing sound. This sound helps to both slow the breath down and to focus awareness on it to prevent your mind wandering. The sound provides something to latch on to, so that your mind can become stiller. When the sound oscillates, your mind too is oscillating.
3. Afterwards, return to normal breathing for a minute or two.

UJJAYI BREATH BENEFITS

Quietens the brain

Slows and smoothes the flow of breath

Calms the digestion

Standing Pose/Mountain Posture (Tadasana)

Standing firmly and evenly on both legs helps increase your awareness of your body and forms an important foundation for the other asanas.

1. Stand with your feet together, big toes and heels touching.
2. Press the feet down to the floor while stretching your legs upwards. Tighten your kneecaps and pull upwards. Compress your hips and buttocks inwards.
3. With your arms extended by your sides, align your head and spine. Stretch the neck and pull your lower abdomen inwards. Lift your sternum, broadening your chest.
4. Press heels and toes downwards, so that pressure is even. Hold this pose for around 30 seconds.

① Sun Salutation (Surya Namaskara)

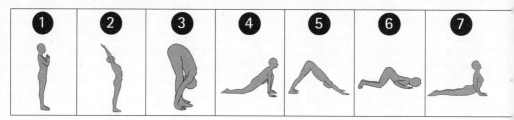

- The Sun Salutation is an important building block in yoga as it combines a number of key poses. For the first Sun Salutation of the day, take a few extra breaths in each pose to allow your body to warm up.
- As you progress through the various phases of the 12-Day Plan, you will find that other key poses are added to your practice.
- Make sure that you do a home-practice every day. The only day you can skip is when you attend a full yoga class. However, some people like to do the Sun Salutation every morning, whether they are planning on going to a class or not – it really helps to set you up for the day.
- There are a couple of variations on the ancient Sun Salutation sequence (version A and version B – see below). Both versions include modifications of the breath.
- This dynamic set of 12 asanas encapsulates the essence of yoga – it's great cardio workout and is effective for toning the body all over.

In its complete form, the Sun Salutation should be done with sequenced breathing (see page 125):

Version A – beginners
Step-by-step technique
1. Bring your hands into prayer pose
2. Inhale. Draw your arms upwards to the sky
3. Exhale, fold forwards
4. Inhale the breath, right leg draws back
5. Exhale to Downward-Facing Dog
6. Hold breath, knees to floor
7. Inhale, Cobra
8. Exhale breath. Downward-Facing Dog

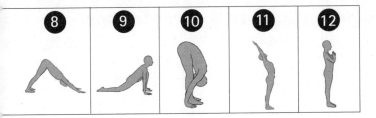

9. Inhale breath, right leg forward
10. Exhale, left foot to left hand
11. Inhale, arms to sky
12. Exhale, hands return to prayer pose.

Version B – intermediate
Step-by-step technique

1. Bring your hands into prayer pose
2. Inhale, Draw your arms upwards to the sky
3. Exhale, fold forwards
4. Hold the breath, right leg draws back
5. Inhale to Downward-Facing Dog
6. Exhale, knees to floor
7. Inhale, Cobra
8. Hold breath, Downward-Facing Dog
9. Hold breath, right leg forward
10. Exhale left foot to left hand
11. Inhale, arms to sky
12. Exhale, hands return to prayer pose.

Practise 12 rounds on either side, alternating your right and left leg. This will help you zip through the rest of the day with a high that is incomparable. And you will find that you can complete 12 rounds (24 sets, meaning 288 asanas!) in 10–15 minutes as you become more physically fit, your metabolism increases for the duration of the day; as does your ability to get toned!

Traditionally, Sun Salutation is best performed outdoors, facing east.

Contraindications and cautions

You should not practise the Sun Salutation if you suffer from high blood pressure, coronary artery diseases, or if you have had a stroke, as it may overstimulate or damage a weak heart or blood-vessel system. You should also be very careful if you have a bad back. If you have a slipped disc or sciatica try a less-vigorous sequence, but take advice from an expert.

Your body should now be sufficiently warmed up for some further poses.

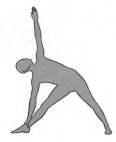

2 Triangle Pose (Trikonasana)

This pose helps to relieve lower back pain and it is an excellent twist for the spine and gut. It stimulates your internal organs, including the liver and gall bladder, and it improves metabolism and circulation through your digestive organs. Whether you are suffering from constipation or IBS, this pose promotes calm within the intestines.

Step-by-step technique

1. Stand in Standing Pose (Tadasana) (see page 127).
2. With an exhalation, step or lightly jump your feet apart.
3. Raise your arms parallel to the floor at the shoulder. Your wrists should be above your ankles, shoulderblades wide, palms down.
4. Turn your left foot in slightly to the right and your right foot out to the right 90 degrees. Align your right heel with the mid-bridge of your left heel. Firm your thighs and turn your right thigh outwards, so that the centre of your right kneecap is in line with the centre of your right ankle.
5. Inhale and extend your torso to the right, directly over the plane of your right leg, exhale, bend from your hip joint, not the waist. Anchor this movement by strengthening your left leg and pressing your outer heel firmly to the floor. Rotate your torso to the left, keeping the two sides equally long. Let your left hip come slightly forward and lengthen your tailbone towards your back heel.
6. Rest your right hand on your shin, the ankle or even the floor outside your right foot. Wherever you choose to place your right hand, make sure that it does not distort the sides of your torso. Stretch your left arm towards the ceiling, in line with the tops of your shoulders. Keep your head in a neutral position or turn it to the left, eyes gazing softly at your left thumb.

Stay in this pose for 6–7 breath cycles.

Contraindications and cautions

- If you have a heart condition, practise against a wall, keeping your top arm on your hip
- If you have high blood pressure, turn your head to gaze downwards in the final pose
- If you have neck problems, don't turn your head to look upwards but continue looking straight ahead and keep both sides of your neck evenly long.

Modifications and props

If you cannot comfortably touch the floor with your bottom hand or fingertips, support your palm on a block or against your shin.

Beginner's tip

If you feel unsteady in the pose, brace your back heel or the back of your torso against a wall.

Benefits

- Stimulates the abdominal organs and improves digestion
- Helps relieve stress
- Stretches and strengthens the thighs, knees and ankles
- Stretches the hips, groins, hamstrings, calves, shoulders, chest and spine
- Relieves backache, especially through the second trimester of pregnancy
- Therapeutic for anxiety, flat feet, infertility, neck pain, osteoporosis and sciatica.

Partnering

A partner can help you learn how to move into this pose properly. Ask them to stand in front of your forward foot, facing you. Inhale your forward arm up, parallel to the floor. Your partner can grasp your wrist and wedge their big toe into your forward hip crease. As you exhale, have your partner pull on your arm and push into your hip crease, stretching the underside of your torso.

③ Revolved Three-angle or Triangle Posture (Parivritti Trikonasana)

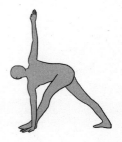

The benefits of the Revolved Triangle are similar to the Triangle, but are even more potent. Though this pose may be difficult it is excellent at stimulating the liver in its cleansing and detoxification function as well as stimulating all the internal organs and regulating digestion. In Revolved Triangle (with head blacked out in the diagram/chart) there is a twist and forward extention, as well as balancing qualities, whereas Triangle Pose is a straightforward side extension.

Step-by-step technique

1. Stand in Standing Pose (Tadasana) (see page 127).
2. On an exhalation, step or lightly jump your feet apart.
3. Raise your arms parallel to the floor at the shoulder. Your wrists should be above your ankles, shoulderblades wide, palms down.
4. Turn your left foot in 45 to 60 degrees to the right and your right foot out to the right 90 degrees. Align your right heel with your left heel. Firm your thighs and turn your right thigh outwards, so that the centre of your right kneecap is in line with the centre of the nipple band. You may experience some negotiation as you twist your upper body slightly to achieve this position.
5. On an exhalation, twist your torso to the right. As you bring your left hip around to the right, push the left thighbone back and firmly ground your left heel. Extend your left hand and arm as far forward as possible.
6. On an exhalation, turn your torso further to the right and lean forwards over your front leg. Reach your left hand down, either to the outer shin, knee or the floor (inside or outside the foot). You can also use a block positioned against your inner right foot. Allow your left hip to drop slightly towards the floor. You may feel your right hip slip out to the side and lift up towards the shoulder, and your torso hunch over your front leg. To counteract this, press your outer right thigh actively to the left and release your right hip away from your right shoulder. Use your right hand, if necessary, to create these two movements, hooking the thumb into the right hip crease.

If you are a beginner, keep your head in a neutral position, looking straight forward, or turn it to look at the floor. If you are more experienced, turn your head and gaze up at your top thumb. From the centre of your back, between your shoulderblades, press your arms away from your torso. Bring most of your weight onto your back heel and your front hand.

Stay in this pose anywhere from 30 seconds to 1 minute. Exhale, release the twist, and bring your torso back to upright with an inhalation. Repeat for the same length of time with your legs reversed, twisting to the left.

Contraindications and cautions

If you have a back or spine injury, only perform this pose under the supervision of an experienced teacher. Or avoid doing it altogether. Also avoid this pose if you have low blood pressure or suffer from migraines.

Modifications and props

One of the most common problems with this pose is keeping your back heel grounded, which makes the pose very unstable. There are various ways to deal with this. First, you can just work towards pressing through the heel (and open the back-leg groin) even though it's off the floor. Second, you can do the pose with your back heel wedged against a wall, which gives you something to push into. Or, you can raise your back heel on a lift and work to gradually lower the lift until your heel stays on the floor.

Benefits

This pose stimulates the abdominal organs and is good for constipation and digestive problems. It strengthens and stretches the legs, hips and spine, opens the chest to improve breathing, relieves mild back pain, stimulates the abdominal organs and improves your sense of balance.

4 Pranayama (Kapalabhati)

Although strictly speaking a Kriya technique (see also page 68), Kapalabhati is a breathing technique used specifically to promote cleansing. The intake of oxygen makes the blood richer and renews the body tissues, while great quantities of carbon dioxide are eliminated. Kapalabhati massages the internal organs, stimulates digestion and elimination and removes stale air and toxins from the lungs. It energises the central nervous system and brings mental clarity and alertness. This practice also helps to tone the abdominal muscles that support the internal organs.

Step-by-step technique

Kapalabhati is a purely diaphragmatic breath and consists of alternating short, sharp exhales generated by powerful contractions of the lower belly. This allows air to be pushed out of the lungs. In Kapalabhati inhales are spontaneous and generated as automatic responses to the release of the contraction of the diaphragm, which allows air to be drawn back into the lungs.

1. Focus on your lower belly. If you are a beginner and find it hard to isolate and contract this area, cup one hand lightly in the other and press them gently against your lower belly. The only part of your body moving is the diaphragm. Your shoulders stay soft.
2. Quickly contract your lower belly, pushing a burst of air out of your lungs. The belly rebounds to suck air into your lungs.
3. Pace yourself slowly at first. Repeat 10–12 times. Rest for a few seconds before starting the second group of 10 and repeat 10–12 cycles 2–3 times. As you become more adept at contracting and releasing your lower belly, you can increase the number of rounds.

Benefits

- Stimulates digestion and activity of the abdominal viscera, so the exercise can be good for constipation
- Cleanses the sinuses and lungs
- Strengthens the diaphragm, intercostal and belly muscles
- Stimulates the brain with a good supply of oxygen
- Enriches the bloodstream and improves circulation
- Clears the mind.

Contraindications and cautions

- Always practise on an empty stomach
- Make sure you take sufficient pauses to inhale deeply and redress carbon dioxide and oxygen levels
- Take extreme caution if you have high blood pressure or vertigo
- Don't do the exercise at all if you suffer from anxiety, epilepsy, hyperventilation, weak lungs, heart trouble or if you are pregnant
- Stop immediately if you begin feeling dizzy, irritable, angry or in any way uncomfortable.

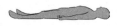

5 Corpse Pose (Savasana)

After you have completed your Sun Salutation asana and Kapalabhati pranayama, remain for 2–5 minutes in Corpse Pose (Savasana).

This pose is good to try at the beginning, middle or end of a session to help you relax, rest, restore, reflect, observe change and counterpose. It helps you to come into the moment and promote inner focus and awareness.

Step-by-step technique

1. Leave plenty of space between your legs so that tension does not build in your hips. Let your feet fall outwards, rotating from your hips. If your feet point upwards you may be holding tension in your calf or thigh muscles. Leave plenty of space between your arms and your upper body. If your arms are too close then your shoulder, back and chest muscles will be too tense. Your fingers should be half-closed: if they are straight or fisted then you will be carrying tension; rotating the palms inwards and outwards will help.

2. Your shoulderblades should soften and fall back onto the floor and your chin should be tucked in towards your chest, creating space in the cervical vertebrae. If your chin is pointing upwards, the cervical vertebrae are constricted and your neck muscles are tense. Place a pillow or blanket under your knees if your lower back is tight. Finally, your facial muscles, eye sockets, cheekbones, lips, jaw and tongue should be soft.

Semi-supine position

This pose is a semi-supine position and an alternative to Savasana. It's good if you have lower back problems.

Step-by-step technique

1. Lie on the mat with your knees bent and your feet placed on the floor, about a hip-width apart. Your knees can either be parted or resting together, if this is uncomfortable. In this pose your spine is resting fully on the floor and your abdomen is relaxed. You might want to try a block under your head to encourage extending the muscles joining the back of your neck to the base of your skull.

2. Place your hands just over your navel and rest your elbows comfortably on the floor to the side. Your tongue should rest on your lower jaw and your throat and face muscles should be relaxed. Your neck is gently lengthened and your chin is tilted slightly forward. Your eyelids should be lowered.

Meditation: put it at the centre of your life

Many people say that meditation is the most powerful and life-changing aspects of the 12-Day Plan, both physically and mentally. The meditation practices are simple techniques, but they are not necessarily easy to do or to incorporate into your life. When you start meditating, setting aside the time to do so requires effort and dedication. But rest assured that incorporating meditation into your life brings you benefits that increase over time. So, remember, when you practise meditation think of it as being like building a deposit account that you can draw on in times of need.

Top meditation tips

- Find a good teacher

  Try to find a meditation class taught by an experienced practitioner; it can really help to learn with others and also to ask questions and get answers from someone who knows the territory.

- Don't meditate on too full a stomach

  Before breakfast is a good time. If you've just eaten, your body is using its energy to digest your food: you are more likely to become sleepy.

- Be realistic about your meditation pose

  Unless you've done a lot of yoga or are naturally flexible, getting into and sitting in a lotus position for 20 minutes may be problematic. However, you don't need to sit in full lotus to meditate. Kneeling on cushions or sitting on a chair is fine. Be as comfortable and upright as you can.

- Make some clear time

  Choose a time to meditate when you really do have a bit of undisturbed time and can relax, even if it's just for five minutes. Turn off your phone. Do what you can to let go of outside demands and take an undisturbed space for yourself.

- Find a quiet place, free from distraction

  If you decide you'd like to meditate regularly, it can really help to sit in the same place each time and create a special atmosphere there, perhaps with a candle, flowers and a picture that inspires you. This does not have to be a large space; the size of a yoga mat will be enough.

- Warm up a little beforehand; chill out a little after

  Prepare to sit with some stretches for the hips and easing out of stiff shoulders, give a bit of kindly attention to any tense places. Finish meditating in time for a cup of tea or just a minute's gazing out of the window before you go on with your day's activities.

- Let go of expectations

  Have faith in yourself and maintain your sense of humour. There are all kinds of meditation experiences, just as there is a huge spectrum of human experience – from serene to grumpy, ecstatic to bored, blissfully clear to distracted. Don't judge yourself as having 'good' or 'bad' meditations. Being aware of whatever is going on is what counts.

- Celebrate your progress!

  Meditation is conducive and supportive of positive change in your life, but be gentle with yourself – you may not become 'enlightened' overnight. Some old habits die hard, but by bringing awareness to them and cultivating an increasingly positive emotional attitude towards yourself, you can achieve great things.

6 Meditation: One to Ten

Meditation occurs when the space in between your thoughts increases. Designate just two minutes on your first day, graduate to three on your second day, then five minutes on your final day.

- Find a comfortable place to sit, on a chair or on the floor
- Allow the natural breath to settle.
- Bring your attention to your navel.
- Observe the gentle expansion of your breath on the inhalation.
- Observe the contraction of the breath back towards your spine on the exhalation.
- Continue to observe the breath without forcing it.

When your mind wanders, as it inevitably will, bring it back to the breath. Count each breath until you get to ten and then begin again at one. Repeat. Make sure that you set a time limit to begin with. You can use a stopwatch if you like.

YOUR NUTRITION

This part of 12-Day Plan is straightforward. Eliminate all of the 'No' foods and introduce foods from the 'Yes' section in The Food Rules chart on page 100.

During the 12-Day Plan we have provide you with a menu guide so you always know what you should be eating. Try the following mouth-watering recipes. There is no need to go hungry when you are avoiding foods like meat, dairy products and gluten-free products. Here are some delicious, filling and comforting recipes for the 12-Day Plan. I have included summer and winter dishes, so there will be plenty to keep you sustained all year round.

The real beauty of the 12-Day Plan menu guide is that all the meals are delicious, easy and quick to prepare. You can save any extra servings to eat the next day. Make sure that you have some good containers in your cupboard, so that you can easily transport your meals into work.

Menu Guide/Days 1–3

Day 1 BREAKFAST
Wheat-Free, Sugar-Free Muesli

4 servings
Preparation time:
10 minutes

This simple recipe has become the mainstay of breakfast mueslis since my India days. It's easy to prepare and can last for ages if you keep it in a good airtight storage container.

Ingredients

100g puffed buckwheat	1 tbsp ground almonds
100g puffed amaranth	2 tbsp raisins or sultanas
100g quinoa flakes	6 chopped dates
1 tbsp sunflower seeds	1 tbsp berries, cranberries, strawberries, raspberries
1 tbsp pumpkin seeds	½ tsp ground cinnamon

Method

Mix all ingredients together in a large storage container with a lid. Serve with oat milk, rice milk, almond milk or water. You can help yourself to it during the 12-Day Plan.

2 servings
Cooking time:
30 minutes
Preparation time:
10 minutes

Day 1 LUNCH
Warm Butternut and Pinenut Salad with Cranberries

This is a tasty salad with a superb balance of texture, taste and colour. It's easy to prepare and very satisfying.

Ingredients

200g butternut squash (peeled, cubed)	175g baby spinach
1 red onion (small, halved and thinly sliced)	40g dried cranberries
2 tbsp cold-pressed virgin olive oil	185g cooked quinoa
¼ tsp cayenne pepper	35g toasted pine nuts

Method

1. Preheat the oven to 220°C. Arrange the butternut squash and onion on an aluminium foil-covered baking sheet and drizzle with 1 tbsp olive oil. Season with the cayenne and pepper, and toss to combine. Roast for 30 minutes or until tender and just beginning to brown.

2. Meanwhile, steam the spinach for 1–2 minutes until bright green and slightly wilted. Drain and squeeze out any excess water.

3. In a large bowl combine the squash, onion, spinach, dried cranberries, quinoa and the remaining tablespoon of olive oil. Season with salt and pepper to taste. Serve warm or at room temperature. Toast pine nuts under a gentle heat and serve.

Day 1 DINNER
Summer Tagine

Definitely worth the wait, this delicious tagine will vanquish all thoughts of being on a detox!

2 servings
Cooking time:
30 minutes
Preparation time:
20 minutes

Ingredients

1kg vine tomatoes, skinned, deseeded and chopped	4 tbsp olive oil
250g green beans, blanched and cut into 2cm pieces	1 tsp cardamom seeds
175g podded broad beans, blanched and peeled to remove tough outer skin	1 tsp ground cinnamon
	2 tsp runny honey
1 medium onion, finely chopped	**To garnish:**
	35g toasted walnuts, chopped
	1 medium lemon, cut into wedges

Method

1. Sauté the onion in 2 tbsp olive oil until soft before adding the tomatoes and spices. Cook gently until the tomatoes start to break up and then add the other 2 tbsp oil and a little water if the sauce seems too thick. Season well.

2. Add the green beans and simmer gently for 15–20 minutes until cooked but still crunchy, adding a little water if necessary.

3. Finally stir in the honey and the broad beans and simmer for a further 5 minutes, at which point the sauce should be quite thick.
4. Serve with a fruity couscous and fresh herbs.

Day 2 BREAKFAST
Cinnamon Fruit Porridge

1 serving
Cooking time:
10 minutes
Preparation time:
10 minutes

This simple breakfast dish is a great alternative to the muesli you've already tried, especially on cold winter mornings.

Ingredients
80g millet and 80g buckwheat flakes or 80g gluten-free porridge oats
1tbsp ground cinnamon
Any fruit, chopped, grated or whole
Handful of mixed seeds such as sesame or pumpkin
Raw organic honey or organic maple syrup
Almond, rice or oat milk

Method
1. Place the oats in a pan and cover with water. Bring to the boil then gently simmer, stirring until the porridge thickens.
2. Sprinkle a handful of mixed seeds, such as sesame, pumpkin, sunflower and linseeds.
3. Add a teaspoon of raw organic honey or organic maple syrup to taste.
4. Serve with almond milk, rice milk or oat milk.

Day 2 LUNCH
Eat leftover Summer Tagine (see page 139) from last night, with:

Beetroot and Pomegranate Salad

2 servings
Cooking time:
30 minutes
Preparation time:
10 minutes

Beetroot and pomegranate? Not an obvious choice, you might think, but this combination is a winner!

Ingredients
3–4 medium beetroots
30g fresh coriander leaves
154g pomegranate seeds
For the dressing:

2–3 tbsp lemon juice
2 tbsp walnut oil
1–2 tbsp toasted sesame oil

Method

1. Steam the beetroots and peel when cooled. Or, better still, try grating them raw.
2. If you have a spiraliser, you can make shoestrings or spaghetti lengths. Otherwise, dice the peeled beets in small cubes.
3. Place the prepared beetroots in a large serving bowl.
4. Whisk the dressing ingredients together in a small bowl.
5. Chop the coriander leaves, add the pomegranate seeds and add to the beetroots.
6. Drizzle the dressing over the salad and gently toss to mix.

Day 2 DINNER
Gluten-Free Mushroom 'Barley' Soup with Buckwheat

This is a wonderfully hearty and healthy soup, which does not make you feel tired and lethargic afterwards, unlike most gluten-based soups.

2 servings
Cooking time:
30 minutes
Preparation time:
10 minutes

Raw buckwheat works as a replacement for many different types of grains, and in this case it works well as a replacement for barley.

Ingredients

2 tbsp olive oil
1 large onion
3 carrots
50g celery leaves
180g fresh mushrooms
1 litre (1¾ pint) bouillion powder

80g untoasted buckwheat (light green/tan colour, not brown)
2–3 bay leaves
½–1 tsp garlic powder
Pepper

Method

1. Heat the oil.
2. Chop the onions.
3. Sauté the onions in the oil until starting to brown.
4. Dice the carrots finely, and add them to the onions. Sauté until starting to soften.
5. Add the mushrooms and sauté a few minutes.
6. Add the rest of the ingredients, bring to a boil, and then simmer until everything is fully cooked and soft.
7. Adjust salt and/or pepper to taste.

Day 3 BREAKFAST
Gluten-Free Bircher-Style Muesli

1 serving
Preparation time:
20 minutes

I just love this breakfast. I had to get into the habit of remembering to soak the nuts and seeds overnight, but once I started it became second nature. It only takes a couple of minutes to put everything into a bowl and fill with water.

Ingredients

6 almonds	1 tsp sunflower seeds
6 pecans	1 small medium apple/pear
1 tsp pumpkin seeds	1 tsp cinnamon

Method

1. The night before soak almonds, pecans, pumpkin seeds, sunflower seeds in a cup and a half of water overnight. Make sure the water is well above the line of the nuts and seeds – they are thirsty and will soak up water overnight
2. In the morning drain off the soaked nuts and seeds and rinse thoroughly until the water runs clear.
3. Place them in your food processor and pulse (start/stop) a few times until the mix starts to break down. 4. Add sliced apple/pear and cinnamon – pulse a few more times until apple/pear is broken into smaller pieces.

Tip the mix into a bowl, add a swish of honey and almond milk and breakfast is done.

Day 3 LUNCH
Avocado and Chicory Salad

1 serving
Preparation time:
20 minutes

Avocado and chicory works wonderfully well together and is absolutely delicious. It's very easy to prepare too.

Ingredients

1 fresh chicory
½ celery stick, chopped
Handful of grapes
½ avocado, sliced
½ apple, chopped

Mandarin slices
50g alfalfa sprouts

Method

1. Tear up the chicory and add the chopped celery.
2. Add the handful of grapes and avocado slices (squeeze over lime to prevent it browning), the apple, mandarin slices and alfalfa sprouts

Day 3 DINNER
Baked Sweet Potato and Borlotti Bean Stew

Sweet potatoes are rich in antioxidant vitamins betacarotene and vitamin E, both of which are required to keep the immune system functioning and to keep the skin in good condition. When topped with the rich, thick bean stew, all thoughts of cleansing will vanish!

2 servings
Cooking time:
45 minutes
Preparation time:
10 minutes

Ingredients

1 large sweet potato	1 large red onion, diced
olive oil	50g mushrooms, sliced
1 tbsp coconut oil or olive oil	200g tomatoes
1 garlic clove, crushed	200g borlotti beans

Method

1. Preheat the oven to 200°C.
2. Pierce the sweet potatoes all over. Rub with oil and place on a baking tray.
3. Cook the sweet potatoes until soft all the way through when pierced with a knife.
4. Meanwhile prepare the stew. Heat the oil in a pan and sweat the garlic and mushrooms and cook for 5 minutes. Add the remaining ingredients and simmer for about 5–10 minutes to allow the vegetables to soften and the sauce to thicken.
5. Open the baked sweet potato and add the stew.

CHAPTER 9

Pre-purification phase/
days 4–6

During this phase you start to introduce some further poses into your Mind Body Cleanse practice. Do all the poses from the Preparation Phase before adding in the new ones explained in this section, using the chart on page 112.

Your checklist
- Follow the nutrition guidelines and try some of the suggested recipes
- Remember to do your Mind Body Cleanse practice
- Do some skin-brushing
- Drink hot lemon water first thing
- Drink freshly squeezed juices
- Drink plenty of water
- Try some gentle stretching
- Get ready for the Power Phase, which comes next, by buying in all you need and see it as treating yourself to three days of healthy calm.

MIND BODY CLEANSE PRACTICE/
THE PRE-PURIFICATION PHASE

PRE-PURIFICATION PHASE

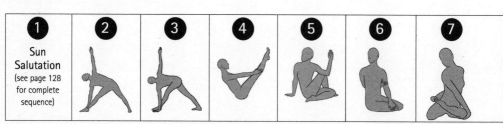

1	2	3	4	5	6	7
Sun Salutation (see page 128 for complete sequence)						

Continue your practice as described in the Preparation Phase/Days 1–3. In this phase we add a couple more poses as well as some new techniques for pranayama and meditation.

Do the following first:

1 Sun Salutation (Preparation Phase, see page 128)

2 Triangle (Preparation Phase, see page 130)

3 Revolved Triangle (Preparation Phase, see page 131)

4 Boat Pose (Navasana)

The Boat Pose improves digestion and strengthens the abdomen, hip flexors and the spine.

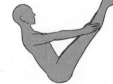

Step-by-step technique

1. Lift through the top of the sternum and lean back slightly. Make sure your back doesn't take up a rounded shape, and continue to lengthen the front of your torso.
2. Exhale and bend your knees, then lift your feet off the floor so that your thighs are angled about 45 degrees to the floor. If you have a history of lower back problems keep your legs bent at the knees.
3. Stretch your arms alongside your legs, parallel to each other and the floor. Draw the inner edges of your shoulderblades in towards each other. Reach through the fingers.
4. Breathe easily. Tip your chin slightly towards the sternum so that the base of your skull lifts slightly away from the back of your neck.
5. At first, stay in the pose for six breath cycles. Gradually increase the time of your stay to 12 breath cycles. Release your legs with an exhalation and sit upright on an inhalation.

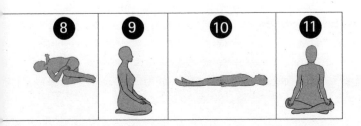

Contraindications and cautions

- Heart problems
- Menstruation
- Pregnancy
- Neck injury: sit with your back near a wall to perform this pose. As you tilt your torso back, rest the back of your head on the wall
- Do not attempt this pose if you have suffered a lower back injury.

Modifications and props

You may find it difficult to straighten your raised legs. If so, try bending your knees and loop a strap around the soles of your feet, gripping it firmly in your hands. Inhale, lean back, then exhale and lift, and straighten your legs, adjusting the strap to keep it taut. Push your feet firmly against the strap.

Beginner's tip

You can prepare for this pose throughout your day without even leaving your chair. Sit on the front edge of a seat with your knees at right angles. Take the sides of the seat with your hands and lean slightly forward. Firm your arms and lift your backside slightly off the seat, then raise your heels slightly off the floor, but not the balls of your feet. Let the heads of your thighbones sink into the pull of gravity and push the top of your sternum forward and up.

Benefits

- Improves digestion
- Strengthens the abdomen, hip flexors and spine
- Stimulates the kidneys, thyroid and prostate glands, and intestines
- Helps relieve stress.

The importance of twists

In this Pre-Purification Phase of the 12-Day Plan we come face to face with the most important group of poses for cleansing and detoxification, namely twists. Twists are key in this process and it is necessary to explore them fully. Practise one of the following seated twists every day during the 12-Day Plan, and for full spinal movement into old age I recommend doing a twist every day for the rest of your life.

Contraindications
If you have a spinal disc injury, consult your doctor before practising twists of any kind.

⑤ Half Lord of the Fish (Ardha Matsyendrasana)

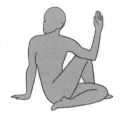

This wonderful twist stimulates the digestive fire in the belly and increases your appetite. The pose massages the liver and kidneys and stretches your shoulders, hips and neck, and energises the spine. It relieves menstrual discomfort, fatigue, sciatica and backache. It is also therapeutic for asthma and infertility.

Step-by-step technique

1. Sit on the floor with your legs straight out in front of you. Using a folded blanket or block under your buttocks is key, especially if you are a beginner or have tight hips.
2. Put your feet on the floor, then slide your left foot under your right leg to the outside of your right hip.
3. Lay the outside of your left leg on the floor.
4. Step your right foot over your left leg and stand it on the floor outside your left hip. Your right knee will point directly up at the ceiling.
5. Exhale and twist towards the inside of your right thigh.
6. Press your right hand against the floor just behind your right buttock and set your left upper arm on the outside of your right thigh near the knee.
7. Pull your front torso and inner right thigh together.
8. Press your right foot into the floor, release your right groin and lengthen your front torso. Lean your upper torso back slightly, against the shoulderblades, and continue to lengthen your tailbone into the floor.
9. With every inhalation, lift a little more through your sternum, pushing your fingers against the floor to help.
10. Twist a little more with every exhalation (a vertebrae or two).
11. Be sure to distribute the twist evenly throughout the entire length of your spine; don't concentrate it in your lower back.
12. Stay in pose for 30 seconds to 1 minute, then release with an exhalation, return to the starting position and repeat to the left for the same length of time.

Contraindications and cautions

If you have suffered a back or spine injury, perform this pose only with the supervision of an experienced teacher.

Benefits

- Stimulates the digestive fire in the belly
- Increases your appetite
- Massages the liver and kidneys
- Stretches the shoulders, hips and neck
- Energises the spine
- Relieves menstrual discomfort, fatigue, sciatica and backache
- Therapeutic for asthma and infertility.

Modifications and props

At first it's often difficult to get your torso to sit snugly against your inner thigh. Position yourself a foot or so away from a wall, with your back to it – the exact distance will depend on the length of your arms. Exhale into the twist and reach back for the wall. Your arm should be almost, but not quite, extended (make sure you aren't sitting too close to the wall, otherwise it will jam your shoulder). Push the wall away and move your front torso against your thigh.

6 Bharadvaja's Twist

This gentle twist is a tonic for the spine and the abdominal organs.

Step-by-step technique

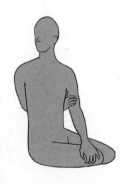

1. Sit on the floor and swing your legs to the left.
2. Lay your feet on the floor outside your left hip, with your left ankle resting in the right arch. Make sure that the pelvis feels even and you are not falling across to your right-hand side. If you are, you can use a block underneath your right hip.
3. Inhale and lift through the top of your sternum to lengthen your front torso. Then exhale and twist your torso to the right from your tummy, keeping your left buttock on, or very close to, the floor. Lengthen your tailbone toward the floor to keep your lower back long. Soften your belly.
4. Place the skin of the knuckles of your left hand to your outer right knee and bring your right hand to the floor in line with your spine

behind you. Always keep the extended arm straight. Pull your left shoulder back slightly, pressing your shoulderblades firmly against your back even as you continue to twist to the right. You can turn your head in one of two directions: continue the twist of your torso by turning it to the right or counter the twist of your torso by turning it left and looking over your left shoulder at your feet.

5. With every inhalation, lift a little more through your sternum, using the push of the fingers on the floor to help. With every exhalation twist a little more from the tummy.

6. Stay in this pose for 30 seconds to 1 minute. Then release with an exhalation, return to the starting position and repeat to the left for the same length of time.

Contraindications and cautions

- Diarrhoea
- Headache
- High blood pressure
- Insomnia.

Modifications and props

For an easier variation of this pose, sit sideways on a chair with the chair back to your right. Bring your knees together and your heels directly below your knees. Exhale and twist towards the chair back. Hold on to the sides of the chair back and lift your elbows up and out to the sides, as if you were pulling the chair back apart. Use the arms to help widen the upper back and move the twist into the space between the shoulderblades.

Deepening the pose

You can increase the challenge in this pose by slightly varying the position of your arms and hands. Firstly, exhale and swing your right arm around behind your back as you twist to the right. If you are able to, take your left arm, just at the elbow, with your right hand; if you can't, hold a strap looped around your left elbow.

Beginner's tip

If you tilt onto the twisting-side buttock (which compresses the lower back), raise it up on a thickly folded blanket. Consciously sink both sitting bones towards the floor.

Benefits

- Improves digestion
- Massages the abdominal organs
- Stretches the spine, shoulders and hips
- Relieves lower backache, neck pain and sciatica
- Helps relieve stress
- Especially good in the second trimester of pregnancy for strengthening the lower back.

Partnering

A partner can help you learn to ground the opposite-side buttock. If you are twisting to the right, have your partner stand to your left side and place his/her hand on the very top of your left thigh.

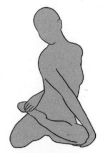

Modifications and props

For an easier variation of this pose, sit cross-legged with your feet underneath your knees, toes pointing forwards. Allow enough space between the pubis and calf muscles to lay a spanned width of your hand in between them. Bring your left hand to the outer side of your right knee and then your right hand back behind your body. Twist from your tummy to the right.

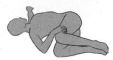

7 Revolved Abdomen Pose (Jathara Parivrtti)

This pose gives a much-needed twist to your intestines, which massages your internal organs and tones your abdominal muscles. It is a wonderful pose to promote bowel movements and relieve constipation, as well as loosen a stiff lower back.

Step-by-step technique

1. Lie on your back on the floor with your arms outstretched from your shoulders, like the letter T, palms facing the ceiling. Let there be a straight line running from your chin to your sternum to your pubic bone.
2. Bend your knees and place your feet flat on the floor.
3. Lift your hips off the floor and swing them to the left.
4. Take your knees toward your chest and drop them towards the floor on the right side of your body.
5. Inhaling, lengthen your spine. Exhale both shoulders towards the floor. Soften your gaze; quiet your hearing. Relax your jaw.

6. Hold the spinal twist for three complete breaths.

7. Lift your legs off the floor and place your feet back down to centre your hips on the floor.

8. Repeat everything to the other side. Repeat this up-down movement on the left side 10 times, or until your waist or back muscles begin to tire.

Focus

In your mind's eye, trace a diagonal line from your right knee to your right hand and then lengthen through the torso along that line. If you feel yourself kinking up in your right waist, place your right thumb in your hip crease and actively draw your right hip away from your shoulder and towards your feet. Then bring your right arm back to its place.

Contraindications and cautions

■ Back or spine injury. Perform this pose only with the supervision of an experienced teacher or avoid it altogether.

Also avoid this pose if you have:
■ Migraine
■ Headache
■ Insomnia
■ Or if you are pregnant.

Benefits

■ Good for sluggish digestion, low energy, stifled breathing and a variety of spinal muscle aches and pains
■ Improves breathing, eases back and neck tension, and soothes frazzled nerves.

8 Cleansing Breath Pranayama

This pranayama exercise is great for clearing negativity from the mind and the body, ventilating the lungs and cleansing the system. It is also known as the Whistle Breath, due to the sound you make while inhaling and the fact that you purse your lips as though you are about to whistle.

You can do this pranayama in either a standing or seated position. For the best results, do this breath at the end of your practice; your asana practice will loosen up any toxins and negativity in the body and this breath will help release them.

Step-by-step technique
Duration: 5 minutes

1. Take a deep breath, hold it for a little while, then purse your lips as if you were going to whistle.
2. Now start exhaling forcefully, little by little, but do not blow the air out as if you were blowing out a candle, and do not puff out your cheeks. They should be hollowed. These successive and forceful exhalations will feel almost like slight coughs, which expel the air until the lungs are completely empty. The effort of the exhalation should be felt in your chest and in your back.

Benefits
- Increased lung capacity
- Stimulates the parasympathetic nervous system
- Increases vitality in the body
- Promotes self-healing and inner calm.

Contraindications
Avoid this breath if you suffer from chronic chills or constipation.

⑨ Meditation (Sankalpa)

Step-by-step technique
1. Coming into a comfortable seat, close your eyes or rest your eyes softly on a single, unmoving point. Invite your body to soften.
2. Turn your palms face up, a gesture of receptivity and openness, resting the backs of your hands on your knees. This meditation is a practice of opening to all that this new 12-Day Plan has to offer.
3. Begin to turn your awareness to your breath, letting it be natural and effortless. The 12-Day Plan is a time of renewal, a time of rebirth. As you stay with your steady, even breath, consider what you are welcoming in as you enter this new phase of light and life in your life. What is the intention you are setting for yourself at this time? Try to capture your intention in a single word, like 'joy' or 'abundance'.

On each inhale, internally and silently say to yourself, 'I am (your intention)'. For example, inhaling, 'I am joyful' or 'I am abundant'. On each exhale, allow your intention to radiate through your body, mind and spirit. When your mind wanders, simply return to this repetition.

4. Continue this meditation for 5–10 minutes. At the end of your practice, allow the repetition to slowly subside. Remain still for a few moments, allowing your breath to deepen, and slowly open your eyes. Give yourself permission to repeat this mantra throughout your day, taking your practice off your cushion and into your life.

There is nothing more radical than the moment you realise that it's possible to reinvent your life. I am not talking about changing your chic look for all-whites and mala beads, or even leaving a regular job to work for the charity of your choice. I'm talking about reconfiguring your mental and emotional attitudes, shifting your vision of life – the kind of inner shift that turns a pessimist into someone capable of seeing the perfection in everything; that lets an angry person channel rage into creative energy; that makes us happier, more peaceful, more in touch with the love and wisdom at our core.

This sort of transformation is the crux of the 12-Day Plan. Yet it's essential to understand what kind of change we're really after, and also to understand what that level of change requires. We don't want to limit our own possibilities by expecting too little from our practice.

Another great practice, and a good alternative to the one above, is Positive Characteristic.

Positive characteristic
As you go through the 12-Day Plan, start paying attention to your mental disposition. Whatever the conscious brain dwells upon, the subconscious mind will bring to fruition. Often our negative self-image can greatly affect our ability to transform ourselves.

Step-by-step technique
1. Take a few minutes to single out a characteristic that would positively affect your life. Try to keep to a single characteristic if possible. It could be compassion, patience, simplicity, decisiveness,

selflessness or non-judgement of others. Sit with this character attribute and think what it would be like to embody this throughout the course of your day. Does the perception of your world change? How will your interactions with those around you change? And are you happier as a result? What other things in your day might change?

2. Return to this image during your day and notice how it changes the tasks and interaction. It takes 12 days to adopt a new mental approach to your life and the life you lead.

YOUR NUTRITION

During the Pre-Purification Phase, we start to streamline our diet in order to condition our body for optimum cleansing during the Power Phase. In warmer months, eat as much raw food as possible.

Menu Guide/Days 4–6

Day 4 BREAKFAST
Berry Breakfast Smoothie

1 serving
Preparation time:
10 minutes

A delicious and simple breakfast smoothie, brimming with antioxidants and flavour!

Ingredients
4 oranges
2 handfuls berries
2 tbsp flax, sesame, sunflower/pumpkin seeds
½ lemon

Day 4 LUNCH

You can finish off the Baked Sweet Potato and Borlotti Bean Stew (see page 143) that you made last night. It will taste even better on the second day: delicious and comforting. And you can try this:

1 serving
Preparation time:
10 minutes

Mixed Salad

A simple tossed salad that will bring out all of the flavours of the leftover Borlotti Bean Stew.

Ingredients

Make a big mixed salad of shredded cabbage and a selection of dandelion leaves, grated beetroot or carrot, watercress, red, yellow or green peppers, half an avocado and spring onions.

Make a dressing, add plenty of finely chopped parsley and sprinkle with sesame seeds and pine kernels.

Day 4 DINNER
Vegetable Quinoa
Nutty, simple, satisfying and delicious!

2 servings
Cooking time:
15 minutes
Preparation time:
5 minutes

Ingredients

50g dried wild mushrooms	1 tbsp tamari
125g quinoa	500ml bouillion powder
175g broccoli, sliced	**To garnish:**
1 tbsp capers	Basil
1 red pepper, chopped	Hempseed oil
2 tbsp gardens peas	Smoked paprika
1 tbsp vegan Worcestershire sauce	

Method

1. Bring the vegetable stock to the boil. Add the dried mushrooms and simmer. Add the quinoa and continue to simmer gently with the lid on for 5 minutes.
2. Add the remaining ingredients, stir and replace the lid and continue to simmer for a further 10 minutes. The quinoa should have soaked up all the water and become light and fluffy – if not, stir and allow to stand with the saucepan lid tightly closed for a further 5 minutes.
3. Serve with green salad or red cabbage. Sprinkle some smoked paprika and chopped basil on top and drizzle with extra tamari and hempseed oil.

Day 5 BREAKFAST

You can have muesli this morning – there shoud be plenty left over, or you can make some more porridge.

Try some Wheat-Free, Sugar-Free Muesli (see page 138) from your storage container.

Day 5 LUNCH
Blackberry, Raspberry and Fennel Salad

Quite delicious! An elegant, light combination of tastes and textures.

4 servings
Cooking time:
10 minutes
Preparation time:
20 minutes

Ingredients

50g walnuts

¼ cucumber

½ fennel, very thinly sliced/shredded

85g watercress, thick stalks removed

1 round green lettuce, washed and dried

150g blackberries, washed and dried

150g raspberries, washed and dried

150g silken tofu

Method

1. Preheat oven to 200°C.
2. Spread the walnuts on a baking tray and put in the hot oven for about 4 minutes until lightly roasted. Remove from the oven and cool.

To make the dressing:

1. Drain the silken tofu by putting it in a bowl lined with kitchen paper and patting dry. Transfer silken tofu to blender.
2. Blend for about 30 seconds until creamy. Put into a bowl ready to serve.

Continue with the salad:

1. Cut the cucumber in half lengthways and then thinly slice to make half-moon slices. Mix these with the fennel and watercress.
2. Arrange whole green lettuce leaves on four plates and pile the cucumber mixture on top. Scatter with the blackberries, raspberries and roasted walnuts and serve, passing the dressing around separately.

Day 5 DINNER
Aduki Bean and Puy Lentil Curry

This wonderful curry recipe was shared by one of my students who had completed the 12-Day Plan.

2 servings
Cooking time:
40 minutes
Preparation time:
10 minutes

Ingredients

1 onion

2 cloves garlic

2.5cm piece ginger

2 sticks celery

1tbsp coconut oil

1tbsp curry powder

1 flat tbsp garam masala

Pepper

4 ripe vine tomatoes

75g aduki beans

75g puy lentils	100g red/orange or yellow pepper
400ml coconut milk	50g sweetcorn
150g kale	50g peas
75g green beans	Serve with brown basmati rice

Method

1. Soften the onions, garlic and ginger together in a little coconut oil. Add the celery. Add the curry powder and garam masala.

2. Add the tomatoes, aduki beans and puy lentils and simmer for 5 minutes or so. Add some pepper and maybe more spices to taste.

3. Add the green beans and peppers. Simmer for 10 minutes or so. Add the kale, peas and sweetcorn. Simmer for 5 minutes.

4. Add the coconut milk and simmer for 5 minutes.

5. While you cook the brown rice, leave the curry on for 10 minutes then turn it off to rest while the rice finishes.

Day 6 BREAKFAST

Orange Spice Granola with Black Mission Figs and Almonds

This recipe is gluten-free, vegan, refined-sugar-free and delicious.

2 servings
Cooking time:
40 minutes
Preparation time:
10 minutes

Ingredients

160g certified gluten-free rolled oats	⅛ tsp ground cloves
50g dried organic figs, sliced	1 pinch ground ginger
50g almonds	Juice from 2 oranges
50g finely shredded unsweetened organic coconut	1–2 tsp orange zest
30g flax seeds	1 tsp maple syrup
1 tsp ground cinnamon	1½ tsp vanilla extract
1/4 tsp ground nutmeg	1 tbsp blackstrap molasses (optional – very distinctive taste)

Method

1. Preheat the oven to 150°C.

2. Line a large baking sheet with parchment paper.

3. Combine all of your dry ingredients: oats, figs, almonds, flax seeds and coconut with all of your spices, in a large bowl.

4. In a small bowl stir together all the wet ingredients: orange juice, zest, maple syrup, vanilla and blackstrap molasses.

5. Pour the wet ingredients over the dry ingredients and stir until well coated to make a granola. Let the mixture sit for 5 to 10 minutes.

6. Spread the granola from the bowl onto the baking sheet(s) and bake for 30–40 minutes. Toss every 10 minutes or so to provide even toasting.

7. Remove from the oven and allow to cool completely – it will become crispier as it cools. Keep in an airtight container.

Day 6 LUNCH
Mixed Salad

1 serving
Preparation time:
5 minutes

This light refreshing salad will tempt you with its peppery flavours and fresh minty tastes.

Ingredients

2 handfuls watercress
Fresh mint
3 spring onions
2 tomatoes
1 red/yellow pepper

3 leaves chicory
125g baby spinach
Bean sprouts drizzled with a lemon
    juice and olive oil dressing

Day 6 DINNER
Spanish-Style Chickpeas with Wilted Spinach and Pine Nuts

2 servings
Cooking time:
10 minutes
Preparation time:
5 minutes

Whether you are doing the 12-Day Plan or not, this detox-friendly recipe is a winning mix of ingredients and tastes.

Ingredients

1 onion
Indian spices of your choice,
    added to taste
¼ tsp ginger, coriander, nutmeg
1 chilli

10 cherry tomatoes, chopped
1 red pepper, chopped
200g chickpeas
200g spinach
Roasted pinenuts, to garnish

Method

1. Cook an onion and add Indian spices of your choice to taste.
2. Add the ginger, coriander, nutmeg and chilli followed by the cherry tomatoes and red pepper.
3. After 10 minutes add the chickpeas.
4. Stir in the spinach at the last minute.
5. Garnish with roasted pine nuts.

CHAPTER 10

Power phase/days 7–9

This is the time during the 12-Day Plan when you really go for it and eliminate those toxins big time!

Well done. You're nearly there. You should be feeling pretty good by now, having spent the last six days absorbing all those simple healthy foods.

Even though this part of the 12-Day Plan is where you will be taking liquids only, you should not feel hungry.

You're only a few days away from feeling totally rejuvenated and energised. Keep going – it will all be worth it!

Your checklist
- Only consume fresh fruit and raw vegetable juices – at least six 300ml glasses per day. This can be in a smoothie or a juice form. In the winter you can make soups for extra sustenance.
- Remember to do your Mind Body Cleanse practice.
- Try some skin-brushing.
- Drink hot lemon water first thing in the morning.
- Drink plenty of water.
- Relax and enjoy the odd nap or two.
- Remember to go for a walk to clear your mind. Meditation is great for clearing the mind too.
- Book yourself a massage and/or go for a steam.
- Try some gentle stretching.
- If you've booked one, go for your colonic hydrotherapy session.

POWER PHASE

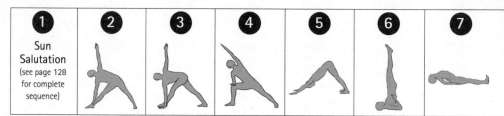

1 **Sun Salutation** (see page 128 for complete sequence)   2   3   4   5   6   7

Continue your practice as described in the Pre-Purification Phase (see page 144). In the Power Phase we add a couple of more poses as well as some new techniques for pranayama and meditation.

Do the following first:

1 Sun Salutation (Preparation Phase, see page 128)

2 Triangle (Preparation Phase, see page 130)

3 Revolved Triangle (Preparation Phase, see page 131)

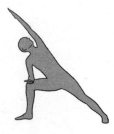

4 Extended Side-Angle Pose (Parsvakonasana)

This pose is great to stimulate the liver and digestive organs as well as the kidneys. Along with all the standing poses, it's great for stability in both mind and body.

Step-by-step technique

1. Standing, bring your feet 3½ to 4 feet apart.
2. Raise your arms parallel to the floor and reach them actively out to the sides, shoulderblades wide, palms down.
3. Turn your left foot in slightly to the right and your right foot out to the right 90 degrees. Align the right heel with the inner bridge of your left heel.
4. Press your left (back) heel to the floor by lifting your inner left groin deep into the pelvis. Then exhale and bend your right knee over your right ankle, so that your shin is perpendicular to the floor. As you

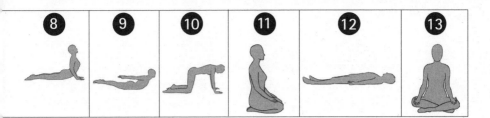

bend your knee, aim your inner knee toward the little toe of your foot. Make sure that your right thigh is parallel to the floor.

5. Lengthen the entire left side of your body. Turn your head to look at your left arm. Release your right shoulder away from your ear. Try to create as much length along the right side of your torso as you do along the left.

Remain in this pose for 6–12 breath cycles.

Contraindications and cautions

- Headache
- High or low blood pressure
- Insomnia.

If you have any neck problems, don't turn your head to look at your top arm. Instead look straight ahead with the sides of your neck lengthened evenly, or look down at the floor.

Benefits

- Strengthens and stretches your legs, knees and ankles
- Stretches your groins, spine, waist, chest and lungs, and shoulders
- Stimulates abdominal organs and helps constipation
- Increases stamina.

Partnering

A partner can help you get a feel for the work of the back leg in this pose. Do the first step. Have your partner stand at your back leg, facing you, and loop a strap around your back inner groin (your partner can also brace your back heel with the inside of one foot). As you bend your front knee, your partner should firmly pull the strap against the inner groin, resisting it opposite to the movement of the front leg. Then, as you lean to the bent-knee side, he/she should continue to pull on the strap, helping you to keep your weight back, on the back leg and heel.

Inversions

Just as the human body has adjusted to an upright position in the course of evolution, it can also learn to perform inversions without any risk or harm. In general, inverted asanas have a drying effect on the pelvic area and abdominal organs, while vital organs such as the heart and lungs are flushed with blood. They are important for the cleansing and detoxification process because of the role they play in stimulating the lymphatic system.

SEQUENCING YOUR INVERSIONS

Shoulder Stand (Sarvangasana) is often done after Headstand (Sirsasana) (although you don't have to do it immediately after), because Sirsasana warms the body up and Sarvangasana cools it down. Additionally, in Sarvangasana the back of the neck is released and the vertebrae are extended, releasing any tension and compression in the neck that an incorrect Sirsasana may have caused. In a well-rounded practice session, Sirsasana should come after standing poses and before other intense work such as backbends and deep twists. If you have neck problems of any kind, it is better to do Sarvangasana before mild backbends because backbends can relieve any tension in the neck caused by Sarvangasana.

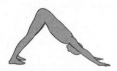

⑤ Downward-Facing Dog (Adho Mukha Svanasana)

Because your heart is higher than your head in this pose, it is considered to be a mild inversion. The flow of blood to the brain also calms the nervous system and can relieve feelings of stress that are often the source of gut-related problems.

Step-by-step technique

1. Come onto the floor on your hands and knees. Set your knees directly below your hips and your hands slightly forward of your shoulders. Spread your palms, index fingers parallel or slightly turned out, and turn your toes under.

2. Exhale and lift your knees away from the floor. At first, keep your knees slightly bent and your heels lifted away from the floor. Lengthen your tailbone away from the back of your pelvis and press it lightly toward your pubis. Against this resistance, lift your sitting bones towards the ceiling, and from your inner ankles draw your inner legs up into your groins.
3. With an exhalation, push your top thighs back and stretch your heels onto, or down towards, the floor. Straighten your knees but be sure not to lock them. Firm your outer thighs and roll your upper thighs inwards slightly.
4. Firm your outer arms and press the bases of your index fingers actively into the floor. From these two points, lift along your inner arms from your wrists to the tops of your shoulders. Firm your shoulderblades against your back, then widen them and draw them towards your tailbone. Keep your head between your upper arms.

Contraindications and cautions
- Carpal tunnel syndrome
- Pregnancy: do not do this pose late-term
- High blood pressure or headache.

Modifications and props
To get a feel for the work of the outer arms, loop and secure a strap around your arms just above your elbows. Imagine that the strap is tightening inwards, pressing your outer arms in against your bones. Against this resistance, push your inner shoulderblades outwards.

Beginner's tip
If you have difficulty releasing and opening your shoulders in this pose, raise your hands off the floor on a pair of blocks or the seat of a metal folding chair.

Benefits
- Improves digestion
- Calms the brain and helps relieve stress and mild depression
- Energises the body
- Stretches the shoulders, hamstrings, calves, arches and hands
- Strengthens the arms and legs

- Relieves headache, insomnia, back pain and fatigue
- Therapeutic for high blood pressure, asthma, flat feet, sciatica and sinusitis.

Partnering

A partner can help you learn how to work your top thighs in this pose. First perform Downward-Facing Dog (see page 162). Have your partner stand behind and loop a strap around your front groins, snuggling the strap into the crease between your top thighs and front pelvis. Your partner can pull on the strap parallel to the line of your spine (remind him/her to extend their arms fully and keep their knees bent and chest lifted). Release the heads of your thighbones deeper into your pelvis and lengthen your front torso away from the strap.

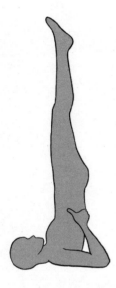

6 Shoulder Balance (Sarvangasana)

Shoulder Stand is a very effective posture when it is practised properly. If you haven't done this pose before I recommend learning it under a teacher's guidance before you try it at home. For our purposes this pose is important in detoxification for its effects, when you are inverted, of bringing the blood back to the heart. This inversion encourages the return of blood through gravity to remove toxins and revitalise the blood.

Step-by-step technique

1. Fold two or more firm blankets into rectangles, measuring about 1 foot by 2 feet, and stack them one on top of the other, or use yoga blocks. You can place a sticky mat over the blankets or blocks to help your upper arms stay in place while you are in the pose.
2. Lie on the blankets with your shoulders supported (and parallel to one of the longer edges) and your head on the floor.
3. Lay your arms on the floor alongside your torso, then bend your knees and set your feet against the floor with your heels close to the sitting bones. Exhale, press your arms against the floor and push your feet away from the floor, drawing your thighs into your front torso.
4. Continue to lift by curling your pelvis and then your back torso away from the floor, so that your knees come towards your face. Stretch your arms out parallel to the edge of the blanket and turn them outwards so that your fingers press against the floor (and your thumbs point behind you).

5. Bend your elbows and draw them towards each other. Lay the backs of your upper arms on the blanket and spread your palms against the back of your torso. Raise your pelvis over your shoulders, so that your torso is relatively perpendicular to the floor. Walk your hands up your back towards the floor, without letting your elbows slide too much wider than shoulder width.

6. Inhale and lift your bent knees towards the ceiling, bringing your thighs in line with your torso and hanging your heels down by your buttocks. Press your tailbone towards your pubis and turn your upper thighs inwards slightly.

7. Inhale and straighten your knees, pressing your heels up towards the ceiling. When the backs of your legs are fully lengthened, lift through the balls of your big toes so that your inner legs are slightly longer than the outer.

8. Soften your throat and tongue. Firm your shoulderblades against your back and move your sternum towards your chin. Your forehead should be relatively parallel to the floor, your chin perpendicular. Press the backs of your upper arms and the tops of your shoulders actively into the blanket support, and try to lift your upper spine away from the floor. Gaze softly at your chest. As a beginning practitioner, stay in the pose for about 30 seconds. Gradually add 5 to 10 seconds to your stay every day or so until you can comfortably hold the pose for 3 minutes. Then continue for 3 minutes each day for a week or two, until you feel relatively comfortable in the pose. Again, gradually add 5 to 10 seconds to your stay every day or so until you can comfortably hold the pose for 5 minutes.

9. To come down, exhale, bend your knees into your torso again, and roll your back torso slowly and carefully onto the floor, keeping the back of your head on the floor.

Contraindications and cautions
- Headache
- High blood pressure
- Menstruation
- Neck injury
- Pregnancy: If you are experienced with the pose, you can continue to practise it late into pregnancy. However, don't take it up for the first time after you become pregnant.

Modifications and props

Rolling up into Shoulder Stand (Sarvangasana) from the floor might be difficult at first. You can use a wall to help you get into the pose. Set your blankets up a foot or so away from the wall (the exact distance depends on your height: if you are taller you will be further from the wall; if you are shorter you will be closer).

1. Sit sideways on your support (with one side towards the wall) and, on an exhalation, swing your shoulders down onto the edge of the blanket and your legs up onto the wall.
2. Bend your knees to right angles, push your feet against the wall and lift your pelvis off the support.
3. When your torso and thighs are perpendicular to the floor, lift your feet away from the wall and complete the pose. To come down, exhale your feet back to the wall and roll down.

Beginner's tip

If you are a beginner you may find that your elbows tend to slide apart and your upper arms roll inward, which sinks your torso onto your upper back, collapsing the pose (and potentially straining your neck). Before coming onto your blanket support, roll up a sticky mat and set it on the support, with its long axis parallel to the back edge (the edge opposite the shoulder edge). Then come up with your elbows lifted on, and secured by, the sticky mat. You can also use a strap around your elbows.

Benefits

- Stimulates the thyroid and prostate glands and abdominal organs
- Improves digestion
- Calms the brain and helps relieve stress and mild depression
- Stretches the shoulders and neck
- Tones the legs and buttocks
- Helps relieve the symptoms of menopause
- Reduces fatigue and alleviates insomnia
- Therapeutic for asthma, infertility and sinusitis.

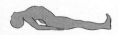 **7 Fish Pose (Matsyasana)**

This is another great pose to lengthen the alimentary canal, and is most often used as an effective counterpose for the shoulder balance.

Step-by-step technique

1. Lie on your back on the floor with your knees bent, feet on the floor. Inhale, lift your pelvis slightly off the floor and slide your hands, palms down, below your buttocks. Then rest your buttocks on the backs of your hands. Be sure to tuck your forearms and elbows up close to the sides of your torso.

2. Inhale and press your forearms and elbows firmly against the floor. Next, press your scapulas into your back and, with an inhale, lift your upper torso and head away from the floor. Then release your head back onto the floor. Depending on how high you arch your back and lift your chest, either the back of your head or its crown will rest on the floor. There should be a minimal amount of weight on your head to avoid crunching your neck. Ninety-five per cent of your weight is passing through your elbows (for more about this, see the Beginner's Tip below).

You can keep your knees bent or straighten your legs out onto the floor. If you do the latter, keep your thighs active and press out through the heels.

Stay for 15 to 30 seconds, breathing smoothly. With an exhalation, lower your torso and head to the floor. Draw your thighs up into your belly and squeeze.

Contraindications and cautions
- High or low blood pressure
- Migraine
- Insomnia
- Serious lower back or neck injury.

Modifications and props
The backbending position in Fish Pose can be difficult for beginners. Perform the pose with your back supported on a thickly rolled blanket. Be sure that your head rests comfortably on the floor and that your throat is soft.

Deepen the pose
To increase the challenge in this pose, slide your hands out from underneath your buttocks and bring them into Salutation Seal (Anjali

Mudra) with your arms outstretched and fingertips pointing towards the ceiling.

Beginner's tip

Beginners sometimes strain their neck in this pose. If you feel any discomfort in your neck or throat, either lower your chest slightly towards the floor or put a thickly folded blanket under the back of your head.

Benefits

- Constipation
- Respiratory ailments
- Mild backache
- Fatigue
- Anxiety
- Menstrual pain.

Partnering

A partner can help you get a feel for the movement of the scapulas in this pose. Perform the pose and have your partner stand straddling your pelvis. They should then lean over and spread their palms on your scapulas, pressing them firmly against your back. But be sure that they don't pull you any deeper into the back bend; they should only support the scapulas against your back torso.

Backbends

In this Power Phase we want to make sure that we keep the bioelectric energy in the body flowing, and backbends are perfect for this.
In backbends, we come face to face with the boundaries of our flexibility, patience and equanimity. But learning to practise within our limitations instead of struggling against them can make backbending an exercise in self-acceptance. Using the breath to control the depth and apex of a backbend offers an interesting encounter with self-acceptance.

If you push too hard or skip ahead to complex backbends without first learning the simple, foundational ones, you run the risk of crunching your lower back, depleting your energy, or even stirring up anxiety. In short, your backbends will not feel melodic or harmonious.

8 Cobra (Bhujangasana)

This gentle backbend opens the heart and lungs, stimulates abdominal organs and helps relieve stress and fatigue.

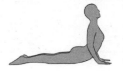

Step-by-step technique

1. Lie flat on your front on the floor. Stretch your legs back, with the tops of your feet on the floor. Spread your hands on the floor under your shoulders.
2. Press the tops of your feet and thighs and your pubis firmly into the floor.
3. On an inhalation, draw your chest upwards. Imagine your upper chest is a sail that has just caught a gust of wind. As you inhale, that sail rises, broadens and floats with ease. Maintain a connection through your pubis to your legs. Press your tailbone toward your pubis and lift your pubis toward your navel. Narrow your hip points. Try not to harden the buttocks.
4. Firm the shoulderblades against your back, puffing your side ribs forward. Lift through the top of your sternum but avoid pushing the front ribs forward, which only hardens the lower back. Distribute the backbend evenly throughout the entire spine.

Hold the pose between 15 and 30 seconds, breathing easily. Release back to the floor with an exhalation.

Contraindications and cautions

■ Back injury
■ Carpal tunnel syndrome
■ Headache
■ Pregnancy.

Modifications and props

If you are very stiff it might be better to avoid doing this pose on the floor. Brace a metal folding chair against a wall and do the pose with your hands on the front edge of the seat, balls of your feet on the floor.

Beginner's tip

Don't overdo the backbend. To find the height at which you can work comfortably and avoid straining your back, take your hands off the floor for a moment, so that the height you find will be through extension.

Benefits

- Strengthens the spine
- Stretches chest and lungs, shoulders and abdomen
- Stimulates abdominal organs
- Helps relieve stress and fatigue
- Opens the heart and lungs
- Soothes sciatica
- Therapeutic for asthma.

Partnering

Your partner can help you learn about the correct action of the pelvis in a backbend. Once in the pose, have your partner straddle your legs. Have your partner bend over and grip the sides of your pelvis, thumbs towards your sacrum, then spread the back of your pelvis, encourage your outer hips to soften, and push your hip points towards each other.

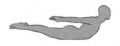

9 Locust (Salabhasana)

This pose is great for toning the kidneys and adrenals as well as cultivating a strong and supple spine. It works the postural muscles of the back to improve the posture and therefore the nervous system and spine.

Step-by-step technique

For this pose you might want to pad the floor below your pelvis and ribs with a folded blanket.

1. Lie on your belly with your arms along the sides of your torso, palms up, forehead resting on the floor. Turn your big toes towards each other to inwardly rotate your thighs and firm your buttocks, so your coccyx presses towards your pubis.
2. Inhale and lift your head, upper torso, arms and legs away from the floor. You'll be resting on your lower ribs, belly and front pelvis. Firm your buttocks and reach strongly through your legs, first through your heels to lengthen your back legs, then through the bases of your big toes. Keep your big toes turned towards each other.
3. Raise your arms parallel to the floor and stretch back actively through your fingertips. Imagine there's a weight pressing down on the backs of your upper arms, and push up towards the ceiling against this resistance. Press your scapulas firmly into your back.

4. Gaze forwards or slightly upwards, being careful not to jut your chin forwards and crunch the back of your neck. Keep the base of your skull lifted and the back of your neck long.

Stay for 30 seconds to 1 minute, then release with an exhalation. Take a few breaths and repeat one or two times more if you like.

Contraindications and cautions
- Headache
- Serious back injury (if you have had a neck injury keep your head in a neutral position by looking down at the floor; you could also support your forehead on a thickly folded blanket)

Modifications and props
If you are a beginner you might have difficulty holding this pose. You can support the area around your lower sternum with a rolled-up blanket to help maintain the lift of your upper torso. Similarly, you can support the front of your thighs with a blanket roll to help support the lift of your legs. Alternatively, you can begin the pose with your hands resting on the floor, a little bit back from the shoulders, closer to your waist. Inhale and gently push your hands against the floor to help lift your upper torso. Then keep your hands in place as you do the pose, or after a few breaths, once you've established the lift of the chest, swing them back into the position described above. As for your legs, you can do the pose with your legs lifted alternately off the floor. For example, if you want to hold the pose for a total of 1 minute, first lift the right leg off the floor for 30 seconds, then the left leg for 30 seconds.

Benefits
- Fatigue
- Flatulence
- Constipation
- Indigestion
- Stress relief
- Lower back pain
- Strengthens the muscles of the spine, buttocks, and backs of the arms and legs
- Stretches the shoulders, chest, belly and thighs.

Partnering

A partner can help you get a feel for the work in the back of the upper arms. Have your partner stand straddling your torso while you perform the pose. They should then lean forwards and press their hands firmly against the backs of your upper arms (triceps). You then push up against this resistance. The partner might also, as they're pressing down on your upper arms, draw the skin away from your shoulders, towards your wrists.

Deepen the pose

If you are at an advanced level you can challenge yourself a bit more with a variation of Salabhasana. Instead of stretching your legs straight back from the pelvis, bend your knees and position the shins perpendicular to the floor. Then, as you lift the upper torso, head and arms, lift your knees as far away from the floor as possible.

Variations

A challenging variation is Makarasana (often translated as 'crocodile' or 'dolphin', but literally 'sea monster'). Your legs are raised in this pose exactly as in Salabhasana, but your fingers are clasped and then your palms are pressed against the back of your head, with your index fingers hooked up underneath the base of your skull. With your upper torso lifted, open your arms out to your sides.

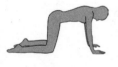 **10** Table Pose (Dwi Pada Pitham)

This pose lengthens the entire line of the gut from mouth to colon. Creating space in the gut like this can help soothe and relieve reflux and bloating.

Step-by-step technique

1. Come into the semi-supine position, feet hip-distance apart.
2. Lift your hips up towards the ceiling. Make sure that your knees stay hip-distance apart during the posture. Stay for six breaths.
3. When you come down, do so slowly, one vertebrae at a time, paying full attention to the spine.

Benefits

- Stretches the chest, neck and spine
- Calms the brain and helps alleviate stress and mild depression

- Stimulates abdominal organs, lungs and thyroid
- Rejuvenates tired legs
- Improves digestion, helps relieve the symptoms of menopause
- Reduces anxiety, fatigue, backache, headache and insomnia
- Therapeutic for asthma, high blood pressure, osteoporosis and sinusitis.

Remember

An asana is not a position that you assume mechanically. It involves a thoughtful process, at the end of which a balance is achieved between movement and resistance.

11 Pranayama: Alternate Nostril Breathing (Nadi Sodhana)

A deeply cleansing and grounding breath that helps to balance emotions, move stagnation out of your lungs, increase lung capacity and purify toxins from the blood.

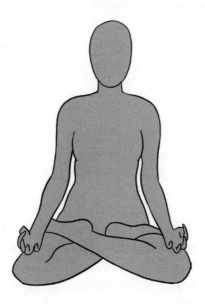

Step-by-step technique

1. Sit in a comfortable seated position and make Mrigi Mudra with your right hand. Use the thumb to close the right nostril and the final two fingers to close the left nostril.

2. Close your right nostril with your thumb. Inhale through your left nostril, then close it with your last two fingers. Open and exhale slowly through your right nostril. Keep your right nostril open, inhale, then close it, and open and exhale slowly through the left. This is one cycle.
3. Repeat 3 to 5 times, then release the hand mudra and return to normal breathing.

Benefits
- Lowers heart rate and reduces stress and anxiety
- Said to synchronise the two hemispheres of the brain
- Said to purify the subtle energy channels (nadis) of the body so the prana flows more easily during pranayama practice.

Contraindications and cautions
Approach the practice of all bandhas and body mudras cautiously, especially if you do not have the direct guidance of an experienced teacher.

12 Savasana
After you have completed the Sun Salutations, rest in Corpse Pose (see page 134) for 2–5 minutes.

13 Meditation
Getting into the Zone
Step-by-step technique
1. Find somewhere to sit, allow your eyes to leaden, and/or listen to some soft, relaxing music or the sound of nature (the real thing or a recording).
2. Remember to keep your straight back as this allows the bioelectric energy to flow through your body. Stay for 5 minutes.
3. Visualise how much better you will feel once you have completed the 12-Day Plan. See yourself with a spring in your step, looking and feeling great – eyes shining, skin clear and vibrant, and your body and mind in a top-notch condition. Most of all, visualise yourself feeling the way you have always wanted to feel, achieving whatever it is that you hope to get out of doing the Cleanse.
4. Remember to congratulate yourself on how far you've come already.

YOUR NUTRITION
What to expect
Now, by consuming nothing but raw, fresh juices for these three days, you give your body a break from normal food and drink. This gives your system a chance to do its own bit of housework, gobbling up unwanted microbes, toxins and matter to leave you feeling rejuvenated and as though you're making a fresh start.

Menu guide/Days 7–9
During the Power Phase you can experiment with which juices and smoothies you take. I always have a smoothie for breakfast during the 12-Day Plan, for lunch I have a juice and for dinner I may even have a soup. This regime changes with the seasons. During spring and summer I may choose something lighter, like a juice, and during the colder months something more warming and filling.

JUICES, SOUPS AND SMOOTHIES
Juices
Juicing lies at the foundation of cleansing and acts to rebuild and rebalance our entire system, delivering vitamins, minerals and antioxidants to the body in an immediate and effective way. Brimming with enzymes and vitality, raw, fresh juice is the most health-affirming, alkalising and rejuvenating food we can take. Most fruits lend themselves to juicing, but the best ones are: oranges, pears, apples, pineapples, lemons, grapefruits, cranberries, strawberries, raspberries, watermelon and pomegranates. Some vegetables are better for juicing than others. I recommend carrots, celery, beetroot, broccoli, cucumber, cabbage, kale, lettuce and fennel. The only rule to remember when juicing is not to combine fruit with vegetables (apart from apples and carrots, which may cross over).

Tips
- When selecting fruit to juice, choose pieces that are almost, but not quite, ripe
- Get into the habit of washing your juicer immediately after use, when it's much easier to clean
- Drink your juices immediately to retain optimum enzyme integrity
- Try adding an ice cube or two for optimum flavour.

ABC of Detox

2 apples
1 beetroot
2 carrots
1cm ginger root

The Great Apple Cleanse

2 apples
2 kale leaves
1 stick celery
1 long cucumber
1cm ginger root

The Green Queen

3 carrots
2 sticks celery
1 bunch watercress
1 large handful spinach
1cm ginger root

Red Carrot Surprise

3 carrots
½ apple
¼ beetroot
1 stick celery
2 large kale leaves
1cm ginger root

Green Goddess

1 bunch fresh parsley
1 handful watercress
8 broccoli spears
2 stick celery
2 large kale leaves
1 long cucumber
1cm ginger root

Broccoli Gone Crazy

8 spears broccoli
3 stick celery
2 pears
1 apple
1cm ginger root

Florida Carrot

3 carrots
½ grapefruit
1 orange
1 small handful mint leaves
1cm ginger root

The Invigorator

2 pink grapefruit
Handful of berries, such as
    strawberries, raspberries and
    blueberries

Stomach Settler

2 carrots
1 pear
½ lemon
1cm ginger root

Zing-a-Zang Apple

3 apples
½ long cucumber
1 small bunch fresh mint
2cm ginger root

Carotene Catapult

3 carrots
1 red pepper
1 spear broccoli
½ sweet potato
1cm ginger root

Belly-Ease Delicious

2 white cabbages
2 fennel bulbs
1 small bunch fresh mint
3 pears
Optional ginger and lime, to taste

Melon Sour

1 melon
Juice of 2 limes
1 stick celery
5–6 mint leaves
2 apples

Summer Healer

3 peaches (or nectarines)
2 handfuls strawberries
1 guava pear

Heaven Scent

1 papaya
2 grapefruit
1 handful of raspberries
Juice of a lime

Sweet Green Melon

1 bunch parsley
¼ white cabbage
½ long cucumber
½ melon

Flat Tummy

¾ papaya
¾ sliced peaches
½ pear, sliced
2 mint leaves
1cm ginger root
Water, to thin

Watermelon Crush

1 small watermelon (the ground-up
    seeds add a nutty and nutritious
    touch)
2 handfuls of berries

Melon Twister

1 melon
Juice of 2 limes
1 stick of celery (remove string)
5–6 fresh mint leaves
2 apples

Skin-Saver

¾ blueberries
¾ pitted cherries
5 strawberries
¼ avocado, peeled and pitted
2 tsp ground flax seed
Water, to thin

Natural Skin-Tanner

160g cantaloupe cubes
160g papaya
Juice 1 orange
120ml carrot juice (or water)
1cm ginger root

Antioxidant Power

75g blueberries
75g raspberries
75g pomegranate kernels
60ml beet juice (optional)
Water to thin

Soups

By far the best way to optimise the effects of your 12-Day Plan is to consume nothing but fresh pressed vegetable and fruit juices. However, in the wintertime you may need some extra sustenance during the Power Phase. Liquidised soups can provide the extra nourishment you may require.

Spinach and Kale Soup

This is a beautiful and satisfying soup, perfect at any time of the year.

4 servings
Cooking time:
30 minutes
Preparation time:
10 minutes

Ingredients

2–3 tbsp extra-virgin olive oil
1 onion, finely chopped
4 cloves garlic, finely chopped
pinch of dried chilli flakes
500g fresh spinach or thawed
   frozen, coarsely chopped

300g fresh kale or thawed frozen, stem
   removed and finely chopped
½ tsp ground nutmeg
1 litre water or bouillion powder
sea salt and freshly ground black pepper,
   to taste

Method

1. Heat the oil in a large saucepan.
2. Add onion, garlic and chili, lower the heat and cook for a couple of minutes or until softened. Stir occasionally.
3. Stir in spinach, kale and nutmeg and gently cook for 1 minute. Then add water or broth and cook for 20 more minutes until the spinach and kale has completely wilted down. Season to taste.
4. Serve as it is or blend it silky smooth, both ways are delicious.

Immortal Carrot and Lentil Soup

Thick and filling, this soup can be kept in the fridge and is ideal for an instant meal. The bright-orange colour shows how rich this soup is in the antioxidant vitamin betacarotene, which will mop up free radicals to prevent them from damaging cells.

4 servings
Cooking time:
40 minutes
Preparation time:
10 minutes

Ingredients

1 tbsp coconut oil, olive oil
2 garlic cloves, crushed
1 onion, roughly chopped
2 large celery sticks, sliced
4 medium-large carrots, sliced
200g red split lentils

Method

Heat the oil in a large pan and sweat the garlic and onion for a few minutes to soften. Add the celery, carrots, lentils, stir, cover with water and bring to the boil.

Cover and simmer for 10 minutes, then blend to your desired consistency.

Sweetcorn Soup

4 servings
Cooking time:
50 minutes
Preparation time:
10 minutes

This dead-simple soup is filled with iron, good vitamins and antioxidants. It is also really delicious and perfect on a cold and rainy day.

Ingredients

4 large sweetcorn cobs, husks removed
1 medium onion, halved and thinly sliced
1 garlic clove, crushed
1 small leek, cleaned and thinly sliced
1 small carrot, chopped
2 tsp lemon juice

½ tsp cumin seeds
½ tsp coriander seeds
1 small, medium-hot red chilli, deseeded and very finely chopped
½ tsp ground turmeric
½ tsp paprika

Method

1. Preheat the oven to 220°C. Lay the sweetcorn, side by side, in a small roasting tin and drizzle with olive oil. Roast in the oven for 30 minutes.
2. Heat the olive oil in a medium pan. Add the onion, garlic, leek and carrot, cover and cook gently for 10 minutes.
3. Meanwhile, heat a dry, heavy-based frying pan over a medium heat. Add the cumin and coriander seeds and shake them around for a few seconds until they have darkened slightly and smell nicely aromatic. Tip them into a spice-grinder and grind to a fine powder. Put into a small bowl with the olive oil, chilli, turmeric, paprika and some freshly ground pepper, then mix. Set aside somewhere cool, but don't chill.

4. Cover and simmer the vegetables for 5 minutes until they are very soft. Add the roasted sweetcorn kernels and simmer a further 3 minutes.
5. Leave the soup to cool, then purée (in batches if necessary) until smooth. Return to the pan and stir in the lemon juice, honey and some pepper to taste.

Cleansing Cold Cucumber Soup
On a hot summer's day this much-beloved soup will help you to think about what might lie beyond the 12-Day Plan.

2 servings
Preparation time:
10 minutes

Ingredients
1 large cucumber, chopped
1 ripe avocado, cubed
2 tbsp red onion, chopped
1 tbsp dill
Juice of ½ lime

Method
1. In a large food processor, combine the cucumber, avocado, red onion, dill and lime juice. Process for 30 seconds.
2. Stream in 1½ cups cold water and blend until smooth.
3. Chill for 30 minutes, or serve immediately and garnish with fresh dill sprigs.

Smoothies
Smoothies make a fantastic and nutritious breakfast. They can include a variety of different ingredients: berries, watermelon, kiwis, pineapple, pears, apricot, cherry, dark grapes, lime, lemon and tangerine. You can add ground seeds too. If you want a thinner, more drinkable smoothie, then you can add one of the following: oat milk, rice milk, water or almond milk We have prepared some smoothie ideas to get you started and to inspire you to create your own favourites. All you need to do is place everything in a blender and blend until smooth.

Superfood Smoothie
450ml unsweetened almond milk
480g baby spinach
150g frozen blueberries
20g superfood greens
4 ice cubes

Hemp Lunch Smoothie

450ml coconut almond milk
480g baby spinach
1 tbsp superfood greens
150g blueberries
2 tbsp hemp powder
1 tsp hempseed oil

Green Sunshine

450ml unsweetened almond milk
480g baby spinach
½ apple
1 tbsp superfood greens
4 ice cubes

Chocolate Avocado Goddess

1 avocado
2 tbsp dark unsweetened cocoa
  powder
2 tbsp agave nectar
4 ice cubes
450ml unsweetened almond milk

Strawberry Coconut Smoothie

150g fresh organic strawberries
300ml organic coconut milk
1 tbsp chia seeds
170ml cold water
1 tsp vanilla extract

Unsweetened shredded coconut for sprinkling on top 'I have lost a staggering 8lb, having been made to feel wonderful as a consequence. I feel so much better in myself, my clothes are looser and I just feel flatter and less bloated. The colonic irrigation has been revelatory and I feel full of energy!'

'My whole attitude to food has now changed and I plan to follow the Cleanse every six months. I now feel great, am much more alert from the moment my eyes open in the morning to the moment they close at night and still can't believe how great I feel.'

CHAPTER 11

Maintenance phase/ days 10–12

Well done! You have completed the Power Phase, eliminating a vast amount of toxic waste and giving your digestive system a full service.

Your eyes should start to look clear and sparkling, your skin glowing, your mind refreshed and your energy levels increased – you will be feeling amazing! During the 12-Day Plan you have not only been removing toxins, waste and unfriendly bacteria from your digestive system, you have also been restoring your internal garden to a state of optimum health and efficiency.

Your checklist
- Remember to do your Mind Body Cleanse practice
- Try skin-brushing
- Drink hot lemon water first thing
- Drink fresh juices
- Drink plenty of water
- Continue to stretch gently.

MAINTENANCE PHASE

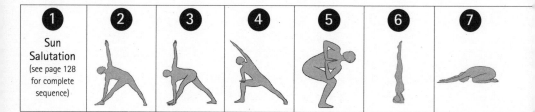

1	2	3	4	5	6	7
Sun Salutation (see page 128 for complete sequence)						

Continue your practice as described during the Power Phase. This week we add a couple of more poses as well as new techniques for pranayama and meditation.

1 Sun Salutation (Preparation Phase, see page 128)

2 Triangle (Preparation Phase, see page 130)

3 Revolved Triangle (Preparation Phase, see page 131)

4 Extended Side Angle Pose/Parsvakonasana (Power Phase, see page 160)

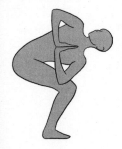

5 Chair Pose and Twist (Utkatasana)

Chair Pose and Twist establishes strength in the gluts, hamstrings, quads and core to create support for the lower back. The revolved variation stimulates the kidneys and adrenals as well as digestion, elimination and liver detoxification.

Step-by-step technique

1. Stand with your feet together, toes and heels touching. Lift your toes and spread them wide. Place each toe back on the floor individually, letting them touch each other as you press them firmly into the floor. From this clear connection to the earth, begin to soften your knees, moving your shins forward as the upper thighs move down and back. Lift your arms up alongside your ears. Rest your gaze on something right in front of you so that your forehead can be soft.

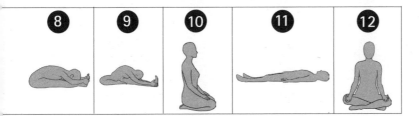

2. Now imagine that you had to stay in this pose for an hour! What changes would you have to make in order to make this happen? Would you release muscular tension? Would you focus on your breath? Ask these questions to help you find an answer.
3. Bring your palms together in front of your chest. Inhale, and as you exhale, twist to the right. On your next inhalation, untwist. Repeat that action, twisting and untwisting twice more. Press your palms together just enough – not too hard – to spread your collarbones. Accept what is available to you today without cranking your arms up. Try to centre your weight on the middle of each foot.
4. Stay here, breathing evenly for a few more breaths, and observe if there is any opening or softening that allows you to twist around more. Inhale to untwist.

Contraindications and cautions
- Headache
- Insomnia
- Low blood pressure.

Modifications and props
You can increase the strength of your thighs by squeezing a block or thick book between them during the pose.

Deepen the pose
Bring the bases of your palms to your thighs and dig your heels deep into the floor. At the same time lift your sitting bones up into your pelvis.

Beginner's tip

To help you stay in this pose, perform it near a wall. Stand with your back to the wall, a few centimetres away from it. Adjust your position relative to the wall so that when you bend into the position your tailbone just touches, and is supported by, the wall.

Benefits

- Stimulates the abdominal organs, diaphragm and heart
- Strengthens the ankles, thighs, calves and spine
- Stretches shoulders and chest
- Improves flat feet.

Partnering

A partner can use either hands or feet to press your heels firmly into the ground.

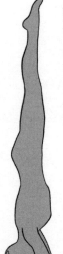

6 Head Balance (Sirsasana)

Head Balance is the king of poses and is considered to be the most important yoga pose of all. The reason for this reputation relates to the effect the pose has on the brain and the lymphatic system. The inversion aspect of this pose causes increased and unrestricted blood flow to the brain, which brings increased oxygen, nutrients and vitality, providing energy for the mind, clarity of thought and ease of concentration.

Step-by-step technique

1. Use a folded blanket or sticky mat to pad your head and forearms. Kneel on the floor. Lace your fingers together and set your forearms on the floor, elbows at shoulder width. Roll your upper arms slightly outwards, but press your inner wrists firmly into the floor. Set the crown of your head on the floor. If you are just beginning to practise this pose, press the bases of your palms together and snuggle the back of your head against your clasped hands. If you are more experienced, you can open your hands and place the back of your head into your open palms.
2. Inhale and lift your knees off the floor. Carefully walk your feet closer to your elbows, heels elevated. Actively lift through your top thighs, forming an inverted 'V'. Firm your shoulderblades against your back and lift them towards your tailbone so that your front torso remains

as long as possible. This should help prevent the weight of your shoulders collapsing onto your neck and head.

3. Exhale and lift your feet away from the floor. Take both feet up at the same time, even if it means bending your knees and hopping lightly off the floor. As your legs (or thighs, if your knees are bent) rise to be perpendicular to the floor, firm your tailbone against the back of your pelvis. Turn your upper thighs in slightly and actively press your heels towards the ceiling (straightening the knees if you bent them to come up). The centre of your arches should align over the centre of your pelvis, which in turn should align over the crown of your head.

4. Firm your outer arms inwards and soften your fingers. Continue to press your shoulderblades against your back, widen them and draw them toward your tailbone. Keep the weight evenly balanced on your two forearms. It's also essential that your tailbone continues to lift upwards towards your heels. Once the backs of your legs are fully lengthened through your heels, maintain that length and press up through the balls of your big toes so that your inner legs are slightly longer than the outer.

5. As a beginning practitioner, stay for 10 seconds. Gradually add 5 to 10 seconds onto your stay every day or so until you can comfortably hold the pose for 3 minutes. Then continue for 3 minutes each day for a week or two, until you feel relatively comfortable in the pose. Again, gradually add 5 to 10 seconds onto your stay every day or so until you can comfortably hold the pose for 5 minutes.

6. Come down with an exhalation, without losing the lift of the shoulderblades, with both feet touching the floor at the same time.

Contraindications and cautions
- Back injury
- Headache
- Heart condition
- High blood pressure
- Menstruation
- Neck injury
- Low blood pressure (warning: don't start your practice with this pose until you are experienced)
- Pregnancy: if you are experienced with this pose, you can continue to practise it late into pregnancy. However, don't take up the practice of Head Balance if you are already pregnant.

Head Balance is considered to be an intermediate-to-advanced pose. Do not perform this pose without prior experience or unless you have the supervision of an experienced teacher.

Benefits

- Tones the abdominal organs
- Improves digestion
- Calms the brain and helps relieve stress and mild depression
- Stimulates the pituitary and pineal glands
- Strengthens the arms, legs and spine
- Strengthens the lungs
- Helps relieve the symptoms of menopause
- Therapeutic for asthma, infertility, insomnia and sinusitis.

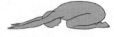

7 Child Pose (Balasana)

Step-by-step technique

1. Kneel on the floor. Bring your big toes together and sit on your heels, then separate your knees to about hip width.
2. Exhale and lay your torso down between your thighs. Lengthen your tailbone away from the back of your pelvis while you lift the base of your skull away from the back of your neck.
3. Lay your hands on the floor alongside your torso, palms up, and release the fronts of your shoulders towards the floor.
4. Child Pose is a great resting pose, and you can stay here anywhere from 30 seconds to a few minutes. Beginners can also use Child Pose to get a taste of a deep forward bend, where the torso rests on the thighs.
5. To come out of the pose, with an inhalation lift upper body from the tailbone.

Contraindications and cautions

- Diarrhoea
- Pregnancy
- Knee injury.

Modifications and props

If you have difficulty sitting on your heels in this pose, place a thickly folded blanket between your back thighs and calves.

Beginner's tip

Child Pose provides us with an excellent opportunity to breathe consciously and fully into the back of the torso.

Benefits

- Gently stretches the hips, thighs and ankles
- Calms the brain and helps relieve stress and fatigue
- Relieves back and neck pain when you do the pose with your head and torso supported.

Partnering

Have your partner place one hand on your sacrum (fingers pointing towards your tailbone) and the other hand on your mid-back (fingers pointing towards your head). As you exhale, your partner can press gently downwards. You can help your partner regulate the pressure on your back.

Variations

To increase the length of the torso, stretch your arms forwards. Lift your buttocks just slightly away from your heels. Reach your arms longer while you draw your shoulderblades down your back. Then without moving your hands, sit your buttocks down on your heels again.

See Half Lord of the Fish (Ardha Matsyendrasana) in the Pre-Purification Phase (see page 147).

8 Forward Bend (Paschimottanasana)

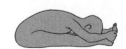

Forward Bends can be wonderfully relaxing and make you feel pleasantly introspective. However, they can also strain or injure your lower back, especially if the backs of your legs are tight. So practise with caution.

This pose stretches the back of your body and compresses the intestine in your lower belly. It is a wonderful pose to stimulate bowel function, relieving bloating, constipation and reflux, and it creates space for all the organs to flow and function.

Gravity and sitting for long periods can cause your torso to compress, which slows down circulation. This pose compresses and then releases the lower belly, creating a flush of fluids to a typically stagnant area of the body. It can really help to get your bowels moving.

Step-by-step technique

1. Sit on the floor with your buttocks supported on a folded blanket and your legs straight out in front of you. Turn your top thighs inwards slightly and press them down into the floor. Press through your palms or fingertips on the floor beside your hips and lift the top of your sternum towards the ceiling as the top thighs descend.

2. Draw your inner groins deep into your pelvis. Inhale and, keeping your front torso long, lean forwards from your hip joints, not your waist. Lengthen your tailbone away from the back of your pelvis. If possible take the sides of your feet with your hands, thumbs on the soles, elbows fully extended; if this isn't possible, loop a strap around your soles and hold it firmly. Be sure your elbows are straight, not bent.

3. When you are ready to go further, don't forcefully pull yourself into the Forward Bend, whether your hands are on your feet or holding the strap. Always lengthen your front torso into the pose, keeping your head raised. If you are holding your feet, bend your elbows out to the sides and lift them away from the floor. Your lower belly should touch your thighs first, and then your upper belly, then your ribs, and your head last.

4. With each inhalation, lift and lengthen your front torso just slightly. With each exhalation release a little more fully into the Forward Bend. In this way your torso oscillates and lengthens almost imperceptibly with the breath. Eventually you may be able to stretch your arms out beyond your feet on the floor.

5. Stay in the pose anywhere from 1 to 3 minutes. To come up, first lift the torso away from your thighs and straighten your elbows again if they are bent.

6. Then inhale and lift your torso up by pulling your tailbone down and into your pelvis.

Contraindications and cautions

■ Asthma
■ Back injury: only perform this pose under the guidance of an experienced teacher.

Beginner's tip

Never force yourself into a Forward Bend, especially when you are sitting on the floor. Often, because of tightness in the backs of the legs, a beginner's forward bend doesn't go very far forward and might look more like sitting up. Be patient.

Modifications and props

Whether you are experienced or not, it's a good idea to sit on a folded blanket in this pose, and if you are a beginner you need to hold a strap around your feet. If you are very stiff you can place a rolled-up blanket under your knees.

Benefits

- Improves digestion
- Calms the brain
- Helps relieve stress and mild depression
- Stretches the spine, shoulders and particularly the hamstrings
- Stimulates the liver, kidneys, ovaries and uterus
- Helps relieve the symptoms of menopause and menstrual discomfort
- Soothes headache and anxiety and reduces fatigue
- Therapeutic for high blood pressure, infertility, insomnia and sinusitis.

9 Head-to-Knee Pose (Janu Sirsasana)

Step-by-step technique

1. Sit on the floor with your buttocks raised on a folded blanket and your legs straight in front of you. Inhale, bend your right knee and draw your heel back towards your perineum. Rest your right foot sole lightly against your inner left thigh and lay the outer right leg on the floor, with the shin at a right angle to the left leg (if your right knee doesn't rest comfortably on the floor, support it with a folded blanket).
2. Press your right hand against your inner right groin, where your thigh joins your pelvis, and your left hand on the floor beside your hip. Exhale and turn your torso slightly to the left, lifting your torso as you push down on, and ground, the inner right thigh. Line up your navel with the middle of your left thigh. You can use a strap to help you lengthen the spine evenly, grounding through the sitting bones.

3. When you are ready, you can drop the strap and reach out with your right hand to take your inner left foot, thumb on the sole. Inhale and lift your front torso, pressing the top of your left thigh into the floor and extending actively through your left heel.

4. Exhale and extend forward from the groins, not the hips. Be sure not to pull yourself forcefully into the forward bend, hunching your back and shortening the front torso. As you descend, bend your elbows out to the sides and lift them away from the floor.

5. Lengthen forward into a comfortable stretch. The lower belly should touch your thighs first, the head last. Stay in the pose anywhere from 1 to 3 minutes. Come up with an inhalation and repeat the instructions with the legs reversed for the same length of time.

Contraindications and cautions

■ Asthma
■ Knee injury: don't flex the injured knee completely; support it on a folded blanket.

Modifications and props

If you can't comfortably reach the extended-leg foot, use a strap. Loop it around the sole of your foot and hold it with your arms fully extended. Be sure not to pull yourself forward when using the strap; walk your hands lightly along the strap while you keep your arms and the front of your torso lengthened.

Beginner's tip

Make sure the bent-leg foot doesn't slide under the straight leg. You should be able to look down and see the sole of your foot. Keep the bent-leg foot active too.

Benefits

■ Calms the brain and helps relieve mild depression
■ Stretches the spine, shoulders, hamstrings and groins
■ Stimulates the liver and kidneys
■ Improves digestion
■ Helps relieve the symptoms of menopause

- Relieves anxiety, fatigue, headache, menstrual discomfort
- Therapeutic for high blood pressure, insomnia and sinusitis

🔟 Pranayama: Bellows Breath (Bhastrika)

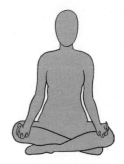

Bellows Breath strengthens and balances the nervous system, bringing peace and tranquility to the mind in preparation for meditation. During Bellows Breath there is an increase in the exchange of oxygen and carbon dioxide into and out of the bloodstream. This action stimulates the metabolic rate, producing heat and flushing toxins and waste out of the body.

Step-by-step technique

1. Sit comfortably in any meditative posture. Sit erect and keep your left hand on your left knee in Gyan Mudra (fold your index and the middle fingers of your right hand to touch the palm).
2. Close your right nostril with your right thumb. Exhale through your left nostril and immediately inhale forcefully. Quickly open your right nostril by closing your left nostril and repeat the procedure.
3. Keep repeating this pattern rapidly, gradually increasing the speed of inhalation and exhalation. Simultaneously contract and expand your abdominal muscles and slowly return to the initial speed.

Contraindications and cautions

- Pregnancy
- Uncontrolled hypertension
- Epilepsy
- Seizures
- Panic disorders
- Avoid practising Bellows Breath on a full stomach.

Beginner's tip

Practise Bellows Breath at a slow breath rate, using a 2-second inhalation and a 2-second exhalation, with no force on inhalation and exhalation. With regular practice the abdominal muscles will become stronger, so the speed can be increased to 30 breaths per minute, using a 1-second inhalation and a 1-second exhalation.

Benefits

- Increases physical vitality
- Clarity of mind
- Activates and invigorates the liver, pancreas, spleen and abdominal muscles, thus toning the digestive system and improving digestion
- Good for the respiratory system including the diaphragm and the bronchial tubes.

11 Savasana

After you have completed the Sun Salutations, rest in Corpse Pose (see page 134) for 2–5 minutes.

12 Meditation

At the beginning and end of your sitting, try to mentally offer thanks to all the people and events in your past who have helped to bring you to where you are, here, now, today. It's an interesting exercise to go on a journey backwards, piecing together the various people you've met, things you've seen or read, or events that have changed the course of your life.

Another interesting meditation to do while cleansing is not to focus directly on yourself, but instead think of others, perhaps less-fortunate people who have yet to be introduced to the benefits and the path that you are now travelling. Meditate on the benefits you may one day be able to bring to such people, when they see the shine in your eyes: the healthier and happier you. Visualise yourself being of assistance to them not by preaching but simply by being yourself. This is the only true and genuine way to help others – to lead by example.

YOUR NUTRITION

What to expect – breaking your fast

'Easy does it!' Make your first meal fresh fruit – just one variety and ideally something in season. Then take it easy regarding food intake: ideally a light diet of fruit and vegetables, plenty of salads, water and juices. Congratulations, you have made it this far!

Day 10 BREAKFAST

Choose your favoured breakfast from the Preparation Phase (see pages 138–42) and the Pre-Purification Phase (see pages 154–7). Enjoy!

Day 10 LUNCH
Super-Boost Sesame Salad

The rich flavour of toasted sesame oil and lemon juice breathe life into this easy-to-make salad without adding any salt or spices.

4 servings
Preparation time:
10 minutes

Ingredients

400g soaked chickpeas
2 celery sticks, finely chopped
6 pieces artichoke heart, roughly
  chopped

6 spring onions, finely chopped
1 tbsp sesame seeds (untoasted)
1 tsp sesame oil or to taste
Juice of ½ lemon

Method

Mix all the ingredients together and serve with salad.

Day 10 DINNER
Squash and Lentil Soup with Chilli and Fennel Seeds

This hearty and subtly aromatic soup is a wonderful soup that will leave you feeling full for hours!

4 servings
Cooking time:
30 minutes
Preparation time:
10 minutes

Ingredients

2 tbsp olive oil
1 onion, finely chopped
2 garlic cloves, finely chopped
2 dried chillies, finely chopped

1 tbsp ground fennel seeds
200g green lentils
1 medium squash, peeled,
  deseeded, cut into 1cm cubes

Method

1. Heat the olive oil in a large pan, add the onion, garlic, chillies and ground fennel seeds, and sweat gently for about 5 minutes.
2. Add the lentils and the diced squash. Cover with water and simmer for about 40 minutes until both the squash and lentils are tender. Season to taste.

3. The soup can be served as it is or you can blend a cupful and stir it back into the pan.

Day 11 BREAKFAST
Choose your favourite breakfast from the Preparation Phase (see pages 138–42) and the Pre-Purification Phase (see pages 154–7). Enjoy!

Day 11 LUNCH
Beetroot and Bean Salad

2 servings
Cooking time:
60 minutes
Preparation time:
10 minutes

This tasty salad is a permutation of the ingredients that are always on my shopping list! Although the cooking time is longer, the results will make it well worthwhile.

Ingredients
4 medium beetroots
200g green or mixed beans, trimmed
40g toasted pine nuts
25g fresh parsley, chopped

2 shallots, finely chopped
4 tbsp extra-virgin olive oil
Freshly ground pepper

Method
1. Preheat oven to 200°C. Line a roasting pan with aluminium foil and place the beetroots inside. Coat them with a tablespoon of olive oil. Roast for about an hour or until tender.
2. Meanwhile, mix shallots with parsley and olive oil. Season with pepper to taste.
3. Bring 1.5 litres of water to a boil. Add the beans and let them cook for about 3 minutes. Blanche the beans rather than cooking them through, so that they stay firm and bright green. Remove the beans from the water and add them to the marinade.
4. Once the beetroots have cooled, slice them as thinly as you like, season with pepper and arrange in a single layer over four large plates. Top with green beans, spooning any leftover marinade on top and sprinkle with toasted pine nuts. Delicious!

Day 11 DINNER
Sweet Potato and Chickpea Casserole
Another heart-warmer, the coriander and cumin in this recipe bring out all
flavours and sweetness in the vegetables.

4 servings
Cooking time: 45
minutes
Preparation time: 10
minutes

Ingredients

1 tsp coriander seeds, crushed

1 tsp cumin seeds, crushed

1 tbsp olive oil

1 red onion, peeled and roughly
chopped into 2cm pieces

2 cloves garlic, finely sliced

1 tsp paprika

2 medium sweet potatoes, peeled
and cut into wedges

400g can chickpeas, drained

400g can chopped tomatoes

2 medium carrots, peeled and cut
into wedges

Flat-leaf parsley, to garnish

Method

1. Crush the coriander and cumin seeds using a pestle and mortar.

2. Heat the oil in a large pan and gently sweat the onion.

3. Add the garlic, crushed spices and paprika and stir until the onions
   are coated.

4. Add the sweet potatoes, chickpeas, tomatoes, carrots and season
   with salt and pepper. Cover. Cook on a low heat for 40–45 minutes or
   until the vegetables are tender.

5. Garnish the casserole with chopped flat-leaf parsley before serving.

Day 12 BREAKFAST
Choose your favoured breakfast from the Preparation Phase (see
pages 138–42) and the Pre-Purification Phase (see pages 154–7).
Enjoy!

Day 12 LUNCH
Chickpeas and Salad

1 serving
Preparation time: 10
minutes

Method

1. Use leftover Sweet Potato and Chickpea Casserole (see page 195)
   served with salad.

2. Make a mixed salad of fresh raw vegetables: celery, grated cabbage, chicory, any green or red salad leaves, chunks of fennel, watercress and any other fresh salad vegetables you enjoy. Make a salad dressing of your choice.

Day 12 DINNER
Beetroot and Chilli Burgers

4 servings
Cooking time: 30
minutes
Preparation time: 10
minutes
Makes 6 large
burgers

A quality veggie burger with all the trimmings can really hit the spot, especially on the last day of the 12-Day Plan. This recipe creates a satisfying burger with a good texture and plenty of flavour.

Ingredients

1 onion, finely sliced	2 cloves garlic, crushed
3 tbsp olive oil	30g sunflower seeds
1 beetroot, grated	150g kidney beans, lightly mashed
½ courgette, grated	30g breadcrumbs
100g vegan Quorn mince (if frozen, thaw first)	½ tsp paprika
½ pepper, finely sliced	1 tsp hot chilli sauce
1 tsp mixed herbs	A splash of Tabasco sauce
	Salt and pepper, to taste

Method

1. Fry the onion in 1 tbsp of olive oil.
2. Place the grated beetroot and courgette onto paper towels and press out as much liquid as you can (this will prevent a soggy burger).
3. In a large bowl, add the rest of the ingredients, except the oil, and season well. The mixture should be fairly dry and easy to press together into burger shapes. If it's still a little wet, add more flour.
4. Place the burgers onto a tray lined with parchment paper and refrigerate for one hour.
5. Carefully place the burgers onto the grill and allow them to cook slowly on a gentle heat. Brush them with a little oil from time to time.
6. Turn after 10 minutes and cook on the other side.

Some final tips

If attaining peace in body and mind was as simple as reminding ourselves to relax whenever we felt agitated, most of us would be blissed out most of the time. Like any other worthwhile skill, though, benefiting from a mind body cleanse takes practice.

The techniques outlined in this book can be a good training ground for cultivating a more peaceful approach to life. The skills we learn in our practice can support us in the rest of our lives, helping us to manage stressful times with clarity and balance.

What can we do to deepen our ability to drop into a state of ease in potentially challenging situations? How can we connect with our inner state of peace when our outer lives are awash with stress and chaos? The techniques we have covered in Part 2 can help you make your way back to balance and tranquility, both on and off the mat. Here are some easy-to-follow tips:

- **Exhale** One of the best ways to bring yourself back down to earth is to lengthen your exhalations. This form of breathing encourages the nervous system to become calm and quiet, moving the body into a more restful state of being.
- **Focus your mind** Sometimes, when the world sends us spinning, we want to do nothing more than drop into an easy chair and stare into space. But this approach often gives the brain free rein to continue its obsessive and agitated thinking. Instead, try focusing your mind in a constructive and engaging way. If you are tired, practise focused relaxation or an absorbing breathing exercise. During your relaxation session, use an eye bag or eye wrap while you're in restorative postures to quiet the eyes and the brain.
- **Minimise external stimulation** Turn off the television, unplug the telephone and dim the lights – turn down the volume of your life, remembering that outer calm nurtures inner calm.
- **Substitute positive thoughts for negative ones** When we are disturbed by negative thought patterns, we can recover our balance by inviting peaceful thoughts into our minds. So the next time you find yourself overcome with an agonising fear or a depressing

thought, notice the negative habit, toss it out, and use your creativity to develop a more positive outlook on the world.

- **Seek out laughter** There's nothing more stress-busting than a first-class belly laugh. Call your funniest friend, or attempt a complicated arm balance that will likely leave you swaying to the floor. Some arm balances are so ridiculously difficult (and let's face it, funny-looking), how could you not laugh?

- **Practise, practise, practise** Like fine wine, equanimity improves over time. Even if you don't happen to feel completely blissed-out in Savasana today, you are priming the body for quiet and ease tomorrow. Repeatedly practising restful postures greases the wheel of relaxation, so you will be able to quickly and easily drop into a deep state of ease further down the line.

- **Steer clear of frozen or tinned vegetables**, which often have added salt and sugar. Also avoid potatoes as they are high in starch and will slow the cleansing process dramatically.

- **Drink** 10–12 glasses of water every day. Drinking plenty of water helps flush out toxins – so ideally you need at least 2–3 litres of filtered water per day.

- **Eat fruit and vegetables with their skins on** – most of the vitamins and minerals are found just beneath the skin (but wash them before you eat them).

- **What you DON'T eat is more important than what you DO eat!**

- **Take snacks with you when you are on the go** and you can also fill up on fresh fruit and fresh juices.

- **Take leftover food from your evening meal to have for lunch the following day** but avoid using a microwave if it needs reheating.

- **Throw away your microwave.** It destroys anything of value in your food!

- **It's important not to drink your calories.** Fruit juice, wine, beer and full-fat lattes all add up to calories that could easily equate to a three-course dinner. Water and green tea are best when it comes to staying hydrated and losing weight.

- **Try to keep portions under control.** Two handfuls of food at a time is more than enough and the vast majority of meals are filling and satisfying if you use nutritious ingredients and chew slowly, thus allowing the 'full' signal to get through and signal to you that you can stop eating.

- **Stock up on snack items** – it's often between-meal, stressed-out hunger pangs that lead to the search for comfort food.
- **For a quick pick-me-up,** treat yourself to a sulphur-free dried fig or fresh high-quality medjool date. As well as naturally satisfying sugar cravings, they have laxative properties to keep things moving inside.
- **For a snack** try pumpkin seeds, olives, hummus and raw vegetables or a rice cake with unsalted hazlenut butter.

Epilogue

After you have completed your first 12-day plan

The 12-Day Plan might be one of the most powerfully purifying endeavours of your life and a truly life-changing experience. On a physical level, when the blood and tissues of the body have been purged of toxins, the body's natural healing mechanisms repair the damage and restore optimal health to your whole system. The effects on other levels of your being are even more profound. Emotionally you are able to let go of a huge amount of baggage as you let go of its physical counterpart. Your energetic levels change and you encourage and attract greater positivity into your life.

Bibliography

Anderson, R., *Cleanse and Purify Thyself* (Christobe Publishing, 2002)

Cruikshank, T., *Optimal Health for a Vibrant Life* (Create Space, 2014)

Desikachar T.K.V., *The Heart of Yoga* (Inner Traditions, 1999)

Edgson, V. and Palmer, A., *GutGastronomy: Revolutionise your eating to create great health* (Jacqui Small, 2015)

Enders, G., *Gut: The inside story of our body's most under-rated organ* (Scribe, 2015)

Feuerstein G., *The Yoga Sutras of Patanjali* (Inner Traditions, 1989)

Iyengar B.K.S., *Light on Yoga: The definitive guide to yoga practice* (Harper Thorsons, 2000)

Knight, R., *Follow Your Gut – the enormous impact of tiny microbes* (TED Books, 2015)

Minger D., *Death by Food Pyramid – how shoddy science sketchy politics and shady special interests have ruined our health* (Primal Nutrition, 2014)

Pedre, V., *Happy Gut – the cleansing program to help you lose weight, gain energy, and eliminate pain* (William Morrow, 2016)

Rauch, E., *Health Through Inner Body Cleaning* (Thieme, 2008)

Reid D., *The Tao of Health, Sex and Longevity* (Simon & Schuster, 1989)

Rosen R., *The Yoga of Breath* (Shambala, 2002)

Satyananda S., *Asana Pranayama Mudra Bandha* (Yoga Publications Trust, 2004)

Recommended supplements

You can buy the following highest quality supplements from my website www.chrisjamesmindbody.com.

'12 Days'
The ultimate 12-day internal cleanse, designed to leave you noticeably more toned, healthier, radiantly alive and glowing with confidence.
• Kickstart your new health regime
• Drop a dress size
• Acquire glowing skin and sparkling eyes
• Achieve mental clarity.

'3R Cleanse'
A condensed cleanse: delicious when added to juices and smoothies.
• Easy to use when you're on the go
• Can be used as a daily fibre supplement
• Increase your energy levels fast.
Recommended intake: 3 sachets daily

'Gorgeous Greens'
Organic daily greens with added enzymes in a unique blend of chlorophyll-rich green foods that can easily be added to water or freshly pressed juices and smoothies.
• Strengthens the immune system
• Helps with bowel regularity
• Defuses free radicals
• Supports your skin to fight ageing.
Recommended intake: 1 sachet daily

'Brilliant Biotic'
The foundation of brilliant health, which begins with a healthy gut.
• 16 viable strains
• 30 billion CFU per serving
• Supports digestive function
• Enhances nutrient absorption
• Assists immune function.
Recommended intake: 2 capsules daily

Active ingredients of Brilliant Biotic:
Lactobacillus acidophilus CUL 60
Lactobacillus acidophilus CUL 21
Bifidobacterium bifidum CUL 20

Bifidobacterium animalis subsp. Lactis 2. CUL-34 2
Lactobacillus salivarius CUL 61
Lactobacillus paracasei CUL 08
Lactobacillus plantarum CUL 66
Lactobacillus casei CUL 06
Lactobacillus fermentum CUL 67
Lactobaciilus gasseri CUL 09
Bifidobacterium animalis subsp lactis CUL 62
Bifidobacterium breve CUL 74
Streptococcus thermophilus CUL 68
Howaru® Lactobacillus acidophilus NCFM™
Howaru® Bifidobacterium lactis HN019
Howaru® Lactobacillus rhamnosus HN001

'Magical Multi'
Anti-ageing from the inside out! Includes a full complement of vitamins
and trace minerals. All wrapped up in heart-healthy coenzyme Q10.
• Rich in antioxidants
• Designed to help defuse free radicals
• Fights off cell oxidation.
Recommended intake: 2 capsules daily

'Hello Aloe'
Inner leaf aloe vera gel is unique because of its concentration and purity. It can be
used topically. Fantastically rich cocktail of vitamins, minerals and trace elements,
and antioxidants.
• Helps with regularity
• Increases protein absorption
• Decreases the amount of unfriendly bacteria and yeast in the gut
• Increases collagen synthesis and skin elasticity.
Recommended intake: 8 drops per day, to be taken and mixed with 100ml water or
used topically

'Buddhi Bath'
Indulge yourself with this intensely magical experience. A unique blend of
penetrating Himalayan salt and detoxifying organic essential oils
• Softens your skin
• Soothes tired muscles
• Replenishes and rejuvenates your mind, body and spirit.
Not for consumption. Avoid contact with eyes

Author's acknowledgements

Firstly, I would like to thank Fiona, my beautiful wife, without whose constant love-bombing and support this book would not have materialised. You are my girl.

I would like to thank my publishers at Vermilion, and wholeheartedly to Morwenna Loughman for your unwavering belief in me. A huge thanks to my gifted editor, Jo Godfrey Wood, who shared my passion in this book and patiently gave structure to it; without you this book would not exist.

Most importantly I would like to thank the great teachers in my life. *Mind Body Cleanse* is a journey that started its life in a classroom at Churcher's College in Petersfield, Hampshire. I would like to thank the late David Pooke, who inspired me to *follow my heart* and read theology at university. And at King's College London, I would like to thank the late Colin Gunton, professor of systematic theology, for his genius mind and for giving me a place. In India T.K.V. Desikachar was the teacher par excellence who taught me how to be a good yoga student. And a special thanks to Fay Beddowes for teaching me so well.

I would like to thank Joy and Adrian Bennett, the Oli Bennett Charitable Trust, and the Prince's Trust for giving me the start that my business needed. I would also like to thank Peter Wright, Richard Cooke, Clive Herbert, and Grace Fodor who helped turn the key.

In my professional life as a teacher, I would like to thank the late David Collins, you are sorely missed, Hermione Crossfield, Panos Kakoullis, – the teacher is oftentimes the student. And to Marcus Cauchi for your humour and your psychiatry!

I would also like to thank my sister, Tania, Neil, Ben and Ella for your love and being the best family I could ever have wished for. Special thanks to my uncle Rodney and Grainne Hedont for being my rock in difficult times.

And finally a special thanks to my friends for their love and support on the way and this is not an exhaustive list: Kim Rudd, Ben Ramalingam, Tony Tregidgo, Giles Parker, Graham Paul, Jim Samuel, Mike Cuomo, Steven Marks, Leon Fisk, Richard and Nicola Marret, Jacqueline Purnell, Anthony Sowyer, Darren Devlin, Charlie Dennis, Pascale Gibon, Marianne Schmidt Barr, Boo and Stan.

And then finally, I would like to thank the Indian gentleman on that train to Kashmir, who pointed at my cigarette and told me, 'This is not yoga!'

Index

Page references in *italics* indicate illustrations.